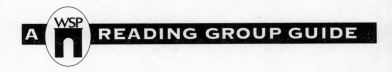
A **WSP** READING GROUP GUIDE

Caroline's Daughters
ALICE ADAMS

ABOUT THIS GUIDE

The suggested questions are intended to help your reading group find new and interesting angles and topics for discussion for Alice Adams' *Caroline's Daughters*. We hope that these ideas will enrich your discussion and increase your enjoyment of the book.

Many fine books from Washington Square Press include Reading Group Guides. For a complete listing, or to read the Guides on-line, visit
http://www.simonsays.com/reading/guides

The
Boston Police Diet
and
Weight Control Program

THE
BOSTON POLICE DIET
and
WEIGHT
CONTROL
PROGRAM

by

SAM S. BERMAN, M.D.

Medical Director, Boston Police Department
Weight Control Program

FREDERICK FELL, INC.

New York

For information address:
Frederick Fell, Inc.
386 Park Avenue South
New York, N.Y. 10016

Library of Congress Catalog Card No. 72-80677

Published simultaneously in Canada by
George J. McLeod, Limited, Toronto 2B; Ontario

Manufactured in the United States of America

STANDARD BOOK NUMBER 8119-0210-2

This book is dedicated
to all unhappy overweights

Acknowledgments

I would like to express my sincere thanks to the Boston Police Department "brass," whose cooperation and red-tape cutting greatly aided in getting the diet and weight control program off the ground, and whose interest has made the Program an on-going thing. Specifically, I would like to mention Police Commissioner Edmund McNamara, Superintendent William Taylor, Superintendent Herbert Mulloney, Superintendent William Bradley, Captain Charles Barry (the liaison officer between the "brass" upstairs and us "plain chickens" below), and Patrolman Frank Hayes, our "notifier" and intermittent loser.

And my thanks to the gentlemen of the Press Room who, when no stories were breaking, came to listen to the inspired stories or alibis of our losers and yes, our non-losers.

Contents

Introduction

IN my more than thirty-five years in the field of medicine, including military service during World War II, I had never been "bitten by the writer's bug." This unbulky literary gem might also have remained in the limbo of unwritten books had it not been for "sincere pressure" from countless numbers of grateful patients . . . and a few friends thrown in. Friends do not usually make good patients, but good patients DO make good friends.

Earlier, I was actually reluctant to add another book to the excessive number of diet books already feeding an insatiable overweight society. But, after discovering that the fast-selling offerings were, in general, cut from the same cloth, and that they were still leaving a residue of millions of unsatisfied, unhappy diet failures, I became convinced that these overweights deserved a better answer to their weight problems. In all modesty, I will admit that I never could accept the conventional explanations given, year after year, regarding the problem of obesity and its proper management.

My own personal beliefs, detailed in this book, have been followed unceasingly for the past twenty-five years by thousands of private patients and are now summed up in a controlled, voluntary project with the Boston Police Department. It should be emphasized that the Program for the Boston Police Department is NO different from those I have prescribed for my private patients over the years. Weight losses and weight control are no strangers to my regular patients. The changing image of the fat policeman prompted newsmen to "pump" the story. Press releases came from the BPD which was deservedly proud of the soon visible achievements, not only on the scale, but to the public's eye.

The Program is now in its eighth year. It supplies a method of healthy eating habits, *and a supplement to correct functional defects*. All this will be explained in the book. As a result of the widespread news interest in this first Police Weight Program, a deluge of mail descended on Headquarters, while many others were delivered directly to my office. The letters were not confined just to the United States; many came from other countries, but each had a constant theme, summed up in one word . . . HELP. These were the multitudes of depressed, disappointed, dejected, semi-starved, exploited overweights, who, according to their letters, had tried everything . . . unsuccessfully.

Each piece of mail was answered. All were informed that the Program was an ongoing one, but that after the first five years the results, plus all operational data, would be made available in book form.

While the factual information about obesity and weight control apply to all, the major target of this book is the "fugitive" from the conventional diets or the "reducing failure" who will have an entirely *new* understanding of his weight problem and what is associated with it. Those who have had the normal metabolism test results will find that the problem does not end with the test itself, but that the trouble actually lies elsewhere. Obesity is not the simple thing it has too long been made out to be. In fact, the problem of obesity is a complex, metabolic, medical disorder . . . not a game to be played with calories and printed diet sheets.

I have no magic formulas up my sleeve. There are NO special inches off or quick loss diets. Gadgetry has no place in the proper management of this serious problem. In short, this is no problem to be entrusted to the hands of the amateurs, commercial or otherwise. The role of your physician is emphasized in cases of excessive weight gain. This entire program is based on getting rid of the excess body fat wherever it has accumulated. The rate or speed of losing is not a governing factor since some lose more quickly than others. The important thing is that THEY ALL

USUALLY LOSE. Very simply, when the weight goes, the inches go and the size decreases. Individuals are not all alike, neither are foods all alike. Some are fattening, others are not. I intend to unmask the calorie and identify it for what it really is . . . just a UNIT of energy and heat . . . and UNITS ARE NOT FATTENING.

I also hope to show you the close association between obesity and aging, particularly premature aging involving early hardening of the arteries, and the all-too-frequent incidence of coronary attacks, stroke, and even diabetes. While mature aging should be accepted as inevitable for all, premature aging should not be, as I intend to show later in this book. While premature aging in some instances may not be stopped, I say that it can be retarded . . . NOT by diets, exercise, and gimmickry, but by supplying a supplement to the vital substance which apparently is insufficiently supplied.

Lastly, this book is not an individual prescription for you or any other reader. Rather, it is a report concerning my own beliefs about the overall problem of obesity, and its strong potential association with the complications of premature aging. It explains why certain persons become fat, while others do not; in fact, cannot. The supplement is described completely . . . why and how I used it, and in particular, how it worked with the Boston Police Diet and Weight Control Program. If you or your physician feel that it might be the key to overcoming your lack of success in losing weight, you can follow the same program in full. The choice is yours.

Sam S. Berman, M.D.
Police Headquarters
Boston, Mass.

The
Boston Police Diet
and
Weight Control Program

CHAPTER I

The BPD Program: What It Means

A PROGRAM FOR ALL OVERWEIGHTS

FAT is fat, and all the rubbing, massaging, rubber belts, rubber garments, electrical currents, appetite suppressors, grapefruit diets, special injections, spot reducers, steam rooms, diuretics, and calorie counters are not going to induce the one condition necessary to lose excess body fat. *This one condition is burning off the fat.*

The members of the Boston Police Diet and Weight Control Program were not just some moderately overweight men who were going on a diet for the first time. Most had been through the mill of conventional restricted calorie diets, those come-ons promising so much, so painlessly. They could be classified as "reducing failures" or "fugitives" from no-eating diets.

Interestingly, my private practice is composed mainly of failures from other methods or groups. This is a strong psychological condition to contend with. I am constantly confronted by desperate, dejected failures, who are thoroughly disillusioned with the so-called "sure" ways to lose weight. Despite the fact that most had been referred to me by others whom I had helped, they actually seemed to dare me to show them something different.

This same challenge was evident when I started the original group of fifty-four men at Boston Police Headquarters in August, 1965. Now I am happy to state, a sincere rapport exists between about four hundred members and myself. I now also know how they felt about the Program when it was first announced. At the time I really didn't know what I was up against.

Policemen are human, no matter what varying opinions have been expressed by their various detractors. Certain ones are just as susceptible to becoming fat as are certain other citizens. They have no special affinity for obesity. It is true, however, that the fat cop is more conspicuous to the citizenry than is the fat fireman or the fat mail carrier or the fat executive or the fat truck driver or the fat doctor. It was for this specific reason that I picked the police for my project. They were subject to the public's daily scrutiny, and I knew that I couldn't hide any failures in the gray mass of anonymity which surrounds the average public. Frankly, I had to have complete confidence in what I was doing and prescribing.

When the BPD communications system sent out the first notices concerning the proposed Program, there was no stampede to enroll. Suspicious comments were made, such as "Who is this doc . . . and is he really a doc" or "What kind of bird food is someone going to want us to eat now?" and, "What's he after . . . no one just gives us something." I can comfortably refer to to all that now, since I have been accepted (I hope).

Still, fifty-four men, generously endowed with protective cushions of fat, did show up the first day. Although their skepticism was very evident, they were courteous and attentive. Screening physical examinations were performed, along with weighing, but it was each man's personal family history that most interested me. I asked about any obesity in either parent, grandparent, or any blood kin. I also asked for any history, immediate or otherwise, concerning the incidence of premature heart attacks, diabetes, stroke, or any diagnosed tendencies towards premature hardening of the arteries, in fact, any aspect of premature aging at all.

Not surprisingly, there was a definite family history of overweights in one branch of the family (sometimes *both*) among most of the men interviewed. This only serves to strengthen an old conviction of mine that *many are literally born to be fat.* This, of course, refers to the potential for becoming fat, as differentiated from the lack of this potential in those who will not and cannot become fat. This statement of fact always brings up the same questions, "Why is what I eat too much for me, but not too much for my partner (or others) who eats even more than I do?" This is the ever-perplexing, sore point with so many unhappy overweights. They are constantly being accused of eating too much without knowing what "too much" is. I had certain never-gains eat the same food as the gainers (even double portions), but the never-gains still did not gain; the gainers did easily.

At the first BPD lecture, the men were shown that all foods are not the same. If you accepted the blanket indictment of "you eat too much," it would imply that *all* foods were the same and that too much of any food would be fattening. Would you believe that you could become fat from eating steak, hamburger, chicken, fish, lettuce, tomatoes or cucumber? Of course not. I also asked for anyone to volunteer that he *never* had intimate relations with such items as pie, cake, cookies, doughnuts, beer, booze, bread, pasta, ice cream, sugared cereals, potatoes, corn, beer, lima beans, and sundry others too numerous to mention. The point was well taken; there were no volunteers. These familiar fattening items are the Carbohydrates. *These* were the real enemy . . . the sugars and the starches, and mainly the sugars such as the refined or commercial products. These are the daily encountered goodies which provide the extra body fat on the overweights. In ordinary circumstances, the mild-mannered natural sugars in fruit and vegetables would be an acceptable source of quick energy. But with our advanced commercialization, there has been a widespread take-over by the *refined* or *commercial* types of sugar which have played a prominent role in the accumulation of excess body fat. Later in the book I will discuss the connection between the misuse of refined sugars and premature aging in those with an hereditary metabolic disorder.

My lecture explained the differences in various foods, their use as *fuel,* and as a source of *repair material.* I also described what foods could and *did* convert to body fat, and *why* they did.

The following excerpts from my lectures will give you a working understanding of why and how individuals become fat and, how to get it off and keep it off. The lecture was and still is a must at each new group enrollment.

Suppose you think of yourself as a machine or engine requiring fuel as the source of the energy. The next step, then, is to activate or utilize the fuel by igniting it. Without being able to ignite fuel, it becomes useless. Upon the efficiency of the igniting system will depend the total amount of fuel which can be utilized. Inadequate igniting will result in less than the full potential from the fuel. Since fuels are *not* all alike, the varying energy and heat output is measured in calories.

QUESTION: What is a calorie?
ANSWER: A calorie is a unit of energy and heat.
QUESTION: Can you become fat from calories? How can you become fat from a unit of energy?
ANSWER: You can't. Only food can convert to fat, and then only certain foods. Of course, just calling something a food or fuel doesn't make it so unless it has calorie value. The more

calories per volume, the more it is a potential source of energy and heat. Being able to *use* this supply of energy and heat depends upon the working of the igniting and utilizing systems. Let's call it the I & U system for easy reference.

QUESTION: What is the I & U system in the body, and where is it?

ANSWER: The *thyroid* gland is the home base from which it secretes the "sparking substance" to help ignite all foods (fuels). One particular food group is not a true fuel. This is the *protein* group. It is actually the repair material from which all the body machinery is made.

If you were going to build a machine engine knowing full well how wear and tear begins as soon as the machine is operational, you would build it from the type of material which would withstand wear and tear the longest. You would use steel, iron, or aluminum and would expect the machine to operate efficiently a reasonable number of years before the wear and tear began to diminish its usefulness.

This same action can be expected from the body material, which is mainly protein. However, a great difference exists in this respect. Our material is LIVING material, and the worn-out cells are cast off or discarded constantly. This means that in order to keep the apparatus functioning efficiently, you would have to keep resupplying the same type of material (protein) daily in amounts equal, at least, to the amount being cast off. This should emphasize to you the vital importance of protein in our daily diet. Without sufficient protein, the body will gradually and inevitably wear out. This is starvation: forcing the body to cannibalize its own protein from the tissues, particularly the muscles.

Now I hope you can understand the danger of any low or restricted calorie diet, in which the total protein had to be reduced in order to keep within the total calorie intake. The less protein, the less efficiently the machinery will function.

QUESTION: What fuels are you talking about? How do we use them for best results?

ANSWER: The two other food groups are *Carbohydrates* and *Fats*. They are as different as coal and wood. Any type of wood is a quick burning fuel and a quick source of energy and heat. So if you depended upon a wood-burning stove to keep your home warm, you would have to keep throwing on wood in order to keep the heat level in the home constant. Well, the carbohydrates act much the same way. They are normally a quick burning source of energy and heat, and if you had to depend upon them as your only fuel, you would frequently have to add them to your own "fire." On the other hand, the fats are like coal. Once you ignite them, the fire will burn longer and hotter. Why? Simply because fats have double the amount of calories potentially contained in the same amount of carbohydrates. Carbohydrates have an energy-heat value of about 4 calories per gram, while the fats have a potential value of slightly more than 9 calories for the same gram. From these figures it would seem logical to take in more fat as the superior fuel. Yes, it would seem so, but why should you when each of you has a generous supply of excess fat piled up on your body.

This pile of fuel is just asking to be ignited and used up. This is the correct way to lose weight: by using up this excess fuel, not by also wasting or starving all other tissues.

QUESTION: How do you ignite and use this piled up fuel? And why haven't I been able to do so, no matter how little I eat?

ANSWER: This is the big question with a big answer. Now, I'll try to explain how the Boston Police Diet and Weight Control Program separates the men from the boys when it comes to satisfactory results. I have already mentioned the thyroid, and that is the source of the "sparking substance" which ignites the fuels and the repair material. The more of this substance that is available, the more fuel which can be fully ignited. Let's say that the thyroid makes the "sparking substance" in that it secretes it, but it still has to be picked up by the blood stream to be carried wherever it has to do its thing. This is the point at which most folks get into trouble.

QUESTION: What kind of trouble? I've had metabolism tests done, and each time they are called normal. Why is this so?

ANSWER: I'm glad you asked. Ninety-five percent, or even more, of all overweights, no matter how much they weigh, will usually come up with normal metabolism test readings. This is a very important but misleading clue. I have seen many grossly overweight persons, who because of these normal readings had been, and are *still* being told, "see . . . there's nothing wrong with your glands . . . you just eat too much."

I sympathize with them, particularly those who really *don't* eat much at all. It's true that the thyroid function appears normal,

*but the trouble does not lie in the thyroid
function.* The trouble lies *between the place
of manufacture* and the *pick-up area.* To put
it more simply, the thyroid is doing its job
normally in secreting the "sparking substance," but something is happening to the
substance *before* it is available for use. I
have seen this happening over the past
twenty-five years, particularly during the
past seven years with the controlled BPD
Program. Here's what happens:

A considerable number of the overweights
develop a form of *self-immunity or self-re-
sistance to their own "sparking substance"
through actual antibody formations. These
antibodies, depending upon the number, will
destroy or neutralize a certain amount of the
spark elements, thus reducing the working
total which survives and becomes actively
available.* To put it simply, the amount of
"sparking substance" secreted is not the
same as the amount that is finally available
for use. You could say that a *block* actually
accounts for the limited spark available, despite the apparently normal metabolic tests.
This deficiency in available spark depends
upon the extent of the antibody formation.
It varies greatly from overweight to overweight. In some, the degree is mild so that
merely limiting the fuel intake is enough to
maintain or even lose some weight. But,
more often, in the heavy heavies, the deficiency is so pronounced that even very small
intake can be too much. Trying to continu-
ally reduce the total food intake by keeping
within a restricted diet also can result in a
heavily restricted protein intake. A step by
step chain reaction occurs. Less protein intake will not repair enough worn machinery

to keep the utilizing factors working efficiently. Not only is there insufficient "spark substance" for full ignition, but also there is too little protein to activate the excess body fat as fuel.

Do you know that there are many three and four hundred pounders who do not lose even on 300 calories daily, yet their metabolism tests are "normal." Certainly these cases can't be accused of eating too much!

For you who have always had a hard time trying to lose on "unhappy diets," and then couldn't keep it off . . . let's do this. I'll put you on *mainly protein,* plus some fresh vegetables and fruit. We'll see what happens. But for the heavy heavies here is something specific. We are going to make up the "sparking substance" deficiency by giving you small amounts of the same substance as a daily supplement, adding it, that is, to what you already have available. This is *not a cure. There isn't likely to be one, since this antibody business is an unwelcome hereditary gift.* This is similar to the hereditary factor in diabetes. The insulin is a supplement, not a cure. The diabetic makes his own insulin, but the amount finally available is inadequate, since apparently there is also a block between the pancreas and the blood stream.

However, by providing this physiological supplement to the spark available, you can actually eat as much protein as you like, providing, of course, you keep away from carbohydrates. Look at it this way. If no carbohydrate is provided by you, then your

excess body fat is the *only* fuel available for
burning. Enough protein is necessary to
keep the burning apparatus (igniting and
utilization) functioning efficiently. Even the
thyroid gland itself is derived from protein.

I encourage such breakfasts as steak and
eggs, hamburgers and eggs, bacon and eggs
(plus other combinations). You need your
energy at the start of each day . . . not at
the close of it. The breakfast must contain
enough protein to activate the entire apparatus in order to start the burning of your
excess body fat for energy. The Supplement
will increase your igniting capacity each time
it is provided.

What you can eat and drink freely and what
you should not eat and drink will be listed
for you.

The first six weeks of the BPD Program became a trial run.
While no one objected to eating steak or hamburger for breakfast, there was strong skepticism among the former calorie counters who had been conditioned to eating small portions of the
food that "doesn't stick to the ribs" in order to lose weight.

Here was the "eatingest" diet they had ever been on. Only
one doubt lingered; "Can you eat like this and still lose weight?"

Th first answer came after the six week period was over. Oh,
this didn't meant that they were through. There's *no such thing
as a six weeks diet.* One learns to eat the right way . . . *permanently.*

The BPD released the first report on the Program's progress at
a press session. The figures and results were most encouraging.
The fifty-four men had lost a total of just over 1,000 pounds.
Those taking the Supplement showed losses up to *three times*

more than those without it. Needless to say, *all* members asked for the Supplement from then on.

When interviewed by the national wire services, the enthusiasm of the losers infected the newsmen, who then created some "complimentary" story headlines such as "Boston Cops Lose Half Ton of Blubber Eating Hamburgers and Taking Little Gray Pill" and "Boston Cops Win Their Losing Battle." I'm sure the police force got the message. When we announced the formation of another group, in addition to the still active original one, there was no lack of candidates. At timed intervals we formed still more groups. I am mentioning these events for a very specific reason. It is only after I was literally overwhelmed with mail from all over the world that I was totally aware of the staggering numbers of dejected, disillusioned, and disappointed dieters, who have literally tried everything. Try to visualize the sudden surge of hope that came over them when reading that fifty-four Boston cops lost a half ton of fat eating hamburgers and taking a "little gray pill." ("Little gray pill" is not exactly a scientific description, but it was the men's own term.)

With so many books and methods on losing weight still appearing on the market . . . and with the usual results . . . the appearance of the BPD Program story caused a general response from the public which all boiled down to one exclamation, "This must be the answer at last." Yes, I believe the answer is in the self-immunity antibody disorder which is a hereditary malfunction.

I cannot see any *specific cure,* but *specific improvement can be had by the proper use of the Supplement . . . plus enough protein intake.* The ban on the useless carbohydrates (those with the empty calories) can be *permanent* so far as I am concerned and so far as your own health is concerned.

The word thyroid when taken out of context can give various false impressions. Many overweight failures, according to letters received, had already been taking even larger doses of a thyroid supplement with no successful results. Even if there had been an actual indication for the large doses, the calorie consciousness led to a serious operational failure. These patients not only had been on therapeutic doses of thyroid, but were also kept on a restricted calorie intake, which invariably meant an inadequate intake of protein.

This combination, unfortunately, would be like speeding up your automobile's engine without increasing the rate of wear and tear on it; it just can't be done. Similarly, here were people taking larger doses of thyroid supplement, which speeded up the metabolism, thereby *increasing the wear and tear of protein tissues, but greatly reducing the re-supply of repair protein.* Only one thing could result from this practice. The deteriorating machinery would lose efficiency, which would in turn affect the whole utilizing apparatus. Very little fuel would then be burned . . . even though it is available as excess body fat.

The BPD Program requires sufficient protein and uses the Supplement in order to keep the higher efficiency operation involved in igniting and burning your excess fat.

Would you believe that instead of cautioning our members not to eat too much, we are more concerned with their not eating enough? It's true! Most dieters are so trained to look for only the lowest calorie items, it becomes difficult to encourage them to shake off the shackles and provide sufficient calories in protein. Of course, those of you who will try to lose weight without the added benefit of the Supplement will have to find your own normal igniting level and then try to keep your protein intake within that particular level. Too little protein can interfere with your full potential to utilize fuel. Your daily wear and tear process must never be ignored or forgotten.

To get back to the Program. At predetermined intervals, new groups were enrolled. Each group underwent the same indoctrination as the first one did . . . with one exception. Through the department grapevine each new member knew about the "little gray pills." It was no longer possible to divide the groups into those taking the Supplement and those not taking it. All clamored for it and would not try to go it with dieting alone. By the way, I just don't like the word diet. It has become synonymous with hunger or not eating. I'd rather say that a person is on a correct eating program since this doesn't seem to imply amounts of food but, rather, kinds of food. Psychologically, it helps to prevent early self-pity.

As more and more police personnel enrolled, we began to make statistical comparisons between their occupational duties. For example, did those who were in cruisers do any better than those who were desk-bound? What about the traffic men? (Very few men who walk a beat are around these days, what with radio and cruisers.) At the start of each session some of the men felt that their results would be better if they could walk more. It didn't take them long to find out that proper eating (along with the Supplement) was more important than worrying about walking or any programmed exercise. Of course, I don't mean to put down walking. I think it is, by far, the best, constant form of daily physical activity. It's still a well-known fact that very few people, if any, actually burn up enough body fat by means of vigorous exercise to make any appreciable difference in their weight. There still have to be dietary changes along with physical activity. Oh, I'm not referring to any temporary weight losses which might occur from heat evaporation (sweating). This weight loss is promptly regained by restoring the fluids lost by sweating. Suffice it to say . . . some of the best losers were among the desk workers.

At this writing, we have completed seven years of the Program. People have asked, "How long does this go on?" The answer is quite simple and to the point. As long as I am able to continue it. There is no specific number of years involved. *Your problem of obesity is a permanent one.* There is little likeli-

hood that one day you are going to find yourself physiologically
changed so that suddenly you can eat and drink anything and
everything with no fear of gaining weight. The never-gains had
this going for them from the beginning. *Do not worry about possible changes occurring later.* Yes, there are persons who apparently remain at a normal weight for years, then at a later period
in life begin to steadily gain weight. These people had the inherent potential from the beginning, but apparently it did not
make enough difference until the "aging" process began to affect
the thyroid center. This now could add up to a noticeable sparking deficiency. The never-gain doesn't gain, no matter what.
Lucky people. That's the difference.

At the end of the first six years some four hundred participants
in the BPD Program had lost a total of approximately 24,000
pounds. This must be understood as a total weight loss peak. It
does not mean that these figures continue constantly and indefinitely. Since the losers were only human . . . and not super-
human . . . a reasonable percentage could be expected to go off
the Program now and then. Not everyone in the Program is, at this
time, at his lowest weight. The majority of them are. Those who
fluctuate a few pounds soon realize how devastating some of the
useless carbohydrate products can be, especially the refined or
commercial sugar ones, on an otherwise satisfactory losing, good
eating, program.

Losing must always be tempered with being able to maintain
the weight. Too many times one sees various commercial weight
losing groups display some big weight losers in a sort of casual
spotlight, but rarely, if ever, does one see the follow-up on those
displayed. Many, many, have promptly regained their lost weight
because, as they put it, "I just couldn't go on indefinitely weighing small portions of the calorie containing foods. . . ."

I should know about these disappointed people. I get many
of them as private rebounds. I just don't seem to see first timers.

All of my private patients, at present, are the failures and fugitives from other diets and groups.

This is no time for modesty. If you not only want to lose weight, but more importantly, keep it off, you will have to realize that people are not alike in various functional performances. The "sparking substance" differs in the total amount available among individuals. If diet alone is to be followed, then the food intake will have to be kept within the individual's own spark availability. If you add the Supplement, you obviously increase the amount of "sparking substance" available each day, and you not only can but should increase your protein intake to promote more active burning of your excess body fat.

THE SELF-IMMUNE HORMONAL BLOCK CONCEPT

With a chapter title like that . . . this could be the beginning of a thrilling science-fiction story. It has been said, "Truth is often stranger than fiction." I'll go along with that because this truth about obesity may very likely come as a jolt to many.

I have never argued with the normal metabolism tests among most of the overweights . . . no matter how much overweight they were. I have had many, many, done on my patients for the past two decades and more. I agree that *most obese persons do not have a glandular condition*. But, I also did not drop the investigation because of that one point. I still could not ignore the often asked question, "Why am I always told that I eat too much . . . and am never believed when I deny eating much at all?" This is usually followed by: "Why doesn't my friend gain . . . when she (or he) eats as much or even more than I do?" These questions were never answered satisfactorily and were usually put off with such vague mumblings as "People are different" or "You really DO eat too much, but you hate to admit it." Big help such remarks can be. I do agree with the statement that people are different; but I would also elaborate on that by adding that *foods are different also. Not all persons can become fat. Not all foods are fattening!* Only when those persons who have the potential to become fat exceed their usable quota of carbohydrates will the excess or unburned fuel (carbohydrate) convert to a reserve pile of fuel . . . and that means extra fat.

Of course, your igniting capacity applies to all foods or fuels. It is not confined to any one group, but only one group can and will convert to fat if unburned. No matter how much igniting or "sparking substance" is secreted or produced in the thyroid, it is still *the amount that is eventually available for use that counts.*

One consistent finding characterized great numbers of the overweights. No matter how normally their thyroid seemed to function (repeated tests bore this out), noticeable discrepancies appeared between the volume of "sparking substance" produced and the volume eventually available for igniting use. The degree of discrepancy varied greatly from individual to individual. In a large number studied, it was so marked that even a small amount of fuel (food) was unable to become fully ignited and burned. Trying to keep the amount of food limited enough to stay within their low igniting capacity meant an abnormally low calorie intake, which in turn meant a poor energy output and virtual near-starvation.

This is precisely why so many unfortunates who plead that they don't eat much should be believed. They can't even ignite and burn very small amounts of food. Who can blame these same persons for quitting diets after a period of unhappy starvation? I can't. I wouldn't relish the daily ritual of weighing out two and three ounce portions of vital food, just for the cause described as a balanced diet. The need for energy is always with us, and even though you have a potential source of energy in the fuel piled on the body (excess fat), this same fuel has to be converted into an active state, requiring igniting and utilizing. Two or three ounces of protein are not going to resupply enough building material to offset the larger amount of worn-out protein tissue cells being cast off. Still, if the available "sparking substance" is limited sufficiently to ignite only the two or three ounce portions of protein, then this is certainly an excellent example for proving the need for the Supplement.

I will say this: if you can lose weight by simply restricting your carbohydrate intake, yet maintain sufficient protein in your daily diet, then apparently your igniting capacity is not very abnormal. But let me press this point: *if it takes starving yourself to achieve sufficient weight loss, the Supplement may well make a big difference* and should be considered for a fair trial. Your physician should cooperate with you in this.

A popular comedian once said that he had the "perfect diet." As he described it, "Eat all you want of everything you want . . . just don't swallow it." While this may be funny, it's no funnier than some radical way-out surgical operations performed on some so-called intractable (unable to lose by any conventional methods) patients. These operations were designed as "shunts," sort of switching the track from the beginning of the intestinal tract to the last portion of the big gut . . . by-passing most of the trackage that does most of the food (fuel) absorption. I think this is, in general, no better than the comedian's "don't swallow" or even the ancient Romans' "vomiting act" which allowed the playboys in togas to eat constantly, then empty the stomach by induced emesis (vomiting, if you please) before the food could be absorbed. This is voluntary starvation . . . hardly to be recommended, as I see it. I won't have to go into the other "benefits" accompanying this type of excess weight prevention, but just bear in mind . . . other things are lost also: vital fluids, electrolytes, vitamins, etc. Speaking of "intractable," I must confess, in all immodesty, that I have yet to see a "non-loser." (I do not refer to the few non-losers who just would not give up their sweets . . . after a fair time. I would firmly suggest they hie themselves elsewhere.) I just

don't believe there is a truly intractable case among individuals
who really want to lose weight. The methods used on non-losers
may have been at fault or the possibility of the self-immune
antibody block was overlooked or unknown. Many of these "in-
tractables" could, in my opinion, have proved tractable had the
Supplement been used.

To summarize:

Obesity is not a simple problem to be treated as an unwanted
stepchild. Not all persons can become obese, no matter how much
or what they eat. Over-eating, per se, can no longer be used as a
convenient catchall term to explain away all obesity problems.

Fuel is the source of energy and heat. All fuels are not alike,
nor are all foods alike. One food group is mainly a tissue repair
material. The calorie is a unit of energy and heat, and the number
of calories in a fuel determines the potential volume of energy
and heat which can be gotten from that particular fuel . . . providing the fuel is fully ignited and utilized. This condition or
proviso is irrevocable.

The fuel with the most caloric value is the source of the most
energy and heat. It depends entirely upon how much of the fuel
is completely used.

The "sparking substance" is secreted or manufactured by the
thyroid gland. It must then be delivered from the gland to the
functional area. Normally, the amount secreted should be the
same as the amount delivered.

Herein lies the trouble. In a great number of overweights, a
discrepancy (varying among different individuals) has been found
to exist between the "sparking substance" secreted and the amount
of this same "sparking substance" that is finally available for use.

This discrepancy is due to a block which exists between the
factory and the pick-up area. This block is caused by an individual's hereditary trait of developing antibodies to his own

"sparking substance." Thus this individual has a self-immune re-
sistance to his own metabolic products.

This is not a disease but a functional metabolic disorder of
hereditary origin. Cure is not likely because there is nothing to
cure. If the volume of "sparking substance" that is available to
the individual shows a sizable deficit compared to the amount
secreted, the individual's igniting and utilizing capacity will be
greatly impaired. In instances of a small deficit, a moderate reduction in the amount of fuel to be ignited may be adequate to
keep within the sparking capacity.

If, however, weight loss is slow, or not forthcoming even with
near starvation diets, I supply a Supplement of the same "sparking substance" for my patients. The results have been demonstrated by the Boston Police Diet and Weight Control Program.

THE FURNACE EXAMPLE

Let's just suppose that some new homes were built by a certain
builder who insisted on the same specifications for each home. He
also provided furnaces which were also identical in specifications.
According to the planning, each furnace had the same fuel potential as the next. Thus, the same amount of coal, if burned
completely, would provide the same heat output for each home.
(Remember, the furnaces were identical in specifications.)

Now, just suppose that at some time, sooner or later, one of
the home owners began to find *incompletely burned coal residue*
in the ashes instead of totally clean ashes. The other furnaces
were completely burning the same amount of coal without a residue of incompletely burned coal. When the furnace experts were
called in to investigate, they were very skeptical, saying that tests
showed nothing wrong with the furnace as compared with the
others. In fact they said, "You are just throwing on *too much*

coal. *Cut down* on the coal." (This sounds familiar, doesn't it.) But *one* question remained unanswered. *Why didn't the other furnaces have the same limitations?* Finally, they admitted that a pattern seemed obvious: certain furnaces (apparently without reason) had this same "functional limitation" which could not apparently be cured or fixed.

The home owner was now told, "If you want your house as warm as the others, and since apparently your furnace won't completely burn up the same amount of coal as the others, you will have to throw on *less coal,* but more often. Unfortunately, you will *always* have to be careful about this."

At about this time another furnace expert spoke up and said, "The fire in any furnace is usually at its lowest by morning, since the last fueling was done the night before. Even under normal circumstances, you would have to be somewhat careful about the amount of coal thrown on the low fire in the morning, but here we have a furnace with a hidden combustion defect, which can prevent even a small amount of coal from being fully ignited. Let me suggest this small but efficient aid. When you go down to the furnace each morning, before you add any coal, *first squirt a small amount of gasoline on the fire.* The gasoline will produce a quick flare-up of flame and, of course, will quickly die down. But at each flare-up, the flame will exceed the normal fire level of the furnace allowing *more coal to become ignited.*"

Let me put this in simpler words. Each time *you* add the gasoline, you are using it as a supplement for the deficient combustibility of the furnace and as such are temporarily making up for the functional defect. Don't forget . . . It's the coal, if completely ignited, that continues to burn . . . not the gasoline. You can squirt some more gasoline (small amounts only) on the fire at noon and again in the late afternoon (5-6 P.M.). The proven value of this type of procedure is that, although you do not cure the functional disorder, you can temporarily make up for the defect by adding the gasoline as a supplement. If you do NOT add the gasoline, for whatever reason, your furnace reverts to its individual normal state.

This is the proven reasoning and operational procedure behind the success achieved with the Boston Police Diet and Weight Control Program, and with several thousand private patients over the past twenty-five years. However, one big difference exists with the overweights. They do not have to throw any coal in the furnace since the fuel is already available as excess body fat. All that is required is to ignite it and to keep the combustion and utilizing apparatus functioning at full efficiency. This means sufficient protein must be supplied, provided it can be utilized. The Supplement will see to that. As long as *no carbohydrate* is supplied, *your excess body fat remains the only fuel available to be ignited and burned.*

Schematic Illustration of Self-Immune Antibody Formation in Obesity Patients

This is particularly significant for those who have great difficulty in losing weight, even on semi-starvation diets, yet show normal metabolism test results.

Also for those who lose slowly and cannot keep it off. This also can apply to most overweights who are more than just a "few pounds overweight."

Thyroid gland is functioning normally (as most tests show). Site of the trouble is in the antibody formation.

If the amount of spark that is finally available (or the amount that gets through) is sufficiently inadequate . . . the Supplement is very definitely indicated. This can make the difference between success and failure.

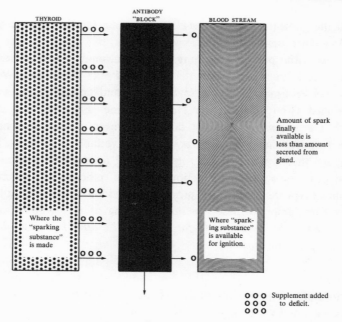

WHY DO PEOPLE BECOME FAT?

The answer is NOT because they eat too much. I know that many of you have been told this so often that you are just fed up with it, especially when you *really don't eat* much.

I believe you, and it is mainly for *you* that this book has been written. Although every person, I believe, could learn something he or she didn't know before, it is the millions of you who have tried everything before, who are going to learn for the first time why they are different. There are always those who can gain and those who cannot and will not gain. These same cannots and willnots, no matter how much they eat of the wrong foods, will still continue to burn off the fuel (food) as fast as it is supplied. (I truly envy them.)

However, if you, the unlucky ones, will only read carefully all that is offered in this book, you not only will learn *why* you gain as you do, but *what you can do about it* . . . logically and sensibly. These two words make all the difference, since no one can deny the fact that there are many ways to lose weight. The question is, *do they make sense?* Always ask yourself, "Can I stay on this particular type of reducing program or method indefinitely . . . and safely?" Herein lies the reason why so many diets fail miserably. You can't continue with them for any reasonable length of time without possibly endangering your health. Although I have faithfully followed my concept for over twenty-five years, the Boston Police Diet and Weight Control Program still stands out as an excellent example of a proven project always open to public scrutiny. You cannot hide mistakes or failures in such openly watched subjects.

To get back to the title of this chapter, "Why Do People Become Fat?" the answer is simply because they take in more of the source of fat tissue than they can possibly use up. Simple, isn't it? It isn't because they eat too much, but because they eat too much of foods that convert to fat. I have already stressed the fact that everyone should have a normal amount of fat cushioning in various parts of the body. But here we are concerned with abnormal fat cushioning. Something does not come from nothing, thus fat isn't produced from nothing. It's always so easy to say, "fat comes from food," but that just isn't enough. What food? All food? The answer is no. Fat results from *one* food group . . . *the carbohydrates.* Normally, fat is an ever-ready reserve supply of fuel, besides being the protective cushion, etc. If this supply of fuel is not used and is allowed to pile up, it just becomes excess fat. The kicker here is: "But why doesn't everyone keep piling up this excess fat?"

Don't mind my repeating certain statements over and over. I cannot overemphasize the importance of your knowing all about your problem before you can really do something about it . . . and in the way it should be done. I have no quarrel with the metabolism tests. I quite agree that the bulk of those performed on many obese persons do show "normal" readings. There is usually no glandular problem, therefore the gland doesn't require treatment. The problem lies beyond the gland itself. One could say that the thyroid gland is doing its job in making and secreting the "sparking substance." However, the amount of this "sparking substance" that is finally available for the igniting function is not always the same as the amount made and secreted by the gland. In more explicit terms, a "block" exists between the factory gland and the body. This block is due to the *antibody formations resulting from the metabolic disorder of self-immunity, which is hereditary in origin and is not a curable condition.*

One can either learn to live with it, if it's not severe, by trying to restrict the total fuel supply to an amount which can be ignited by the individual's spark output. This can be very limited in many, necessitating a very limited intake of food. Unfortunately, this might amount to actual semi-starvation in too many instances, with short-lived weight loss . . . if any. Or the deficit spark factor can be improved on a day to day basis by supplying the same type of substance as a supplement. Don't forget this word supplement . . . not cure, but supplement.

To summarize:

Fat people become fat because their intake of carbohydrates is too much for them.

It cannot be completely ignited and burned because of the deficient "sparking substance."

This deficiency is caused by a functional block (antibodies), which operates between the source of the "sparking substance" (gland) and the area of actual delivery for use.

A daily supplement of this same spark material can favorably change the igniting deficit . . . as long as it is supplied.

This functional block condition is hereditary and usually permanent.

DEFINITIONS OF FREQUENTLY USED DIET WORDS

How many times have you heard your automobile mechanic talk about such mysterious things as camber, torque, displacement, linkage, etc. and wished you knew what he was talking about? You actually didn't want to become an auto expert overnight, but you wanted to have at least a working knowledge about how and where these terms applied to the automobile, as a whole.

I don't expect to give you an overnight course in medicine, either. But to help you understand some of the frequently used words involved in everyday nutrition and diets. I'll try to go lightly over the big ones. I may have to use some of these in order not to lose the complete meaning of some particular subject.

Here are a few . . . and *only* a few . . . since I can't possibly cover everything:

PROTEINS: These are the nitrogen-containing compounds composed of amino acids. These form the basis or the structure of living animal tissue. Although they are widely distributed in nature, they cannot be used by the body in their original form, but must be broken down for utilization by the various digestive juices. This eventually converts them into their usable amino acids.

ENZYMES: This word is all "Greek" to so many persons. Well, why shouldn't it be since it's derived from the Greek words meaning "in yeast." If this still hasn't told you anything . . . then just read on. Enzymes are organic chemical substances which are mostly proteins and are able to change one compound into another by their catalytic action. We are going to use this word enzyme a lot . . . so be prepared for it. In fact, enzymes and digestive juices are going to become quite chummy. They'll be seen and used together throughout this book.

GLYCOGEN: Oh those Greeks! This is another word from the Greek, which somehow means "to produce sweetness." Glycogen is a carbohydrate made in the liver from the simple carbohydrates in your diet. Glycogen is used by the body to break down sugar for energy, and if not completely utilized, acts to increase the synthesis for formation of body fat.

Let me run through a few more of these definitions, then we'll start putting them together in an everyday pattern.

GLUCOSE: You guessed it . . . from the Greek again. It means "sweet." Another name is dextrose. No matter what you call it . . . it's a simple sugar resulting from the breakdown of starch, which itself is another name for liquid glucose. This has been and still is called corn syrup. (It seems that the labels on certain commercial products not wishing to use the word sugar will use less familiar names . . . although they mean the same. It's the "rose by any other name" bit.)

CHOLESTEROL: This one has been the whipping boy in the latest "enemy of the decade" list. Let's just stick to the facts. Cholesterol is from the Greek (what else) and means "bile solids." This is a fat-like, pearly substance found not only in animal fats and oils,

DISCUSSION QUESTIONS

1. Although set in San Francisco, the atmosphere of the book makes the city seem like a small town. Discuss the author's West Coast point of view: is the novel uniquely Californian? Could it have taken place on the East Coast?

2. Would Caroline Carter be considered a good mother or a good wife? After all, she has had five children with three different men. Is she to blame for her daughters' faults or failures?

3. Although Fiona and Jill seem to have the most stable and "important" jobs, by the end of the book, they have both been reduced to joblessness. Discuss how women identify with their jobs and how that identity has changed over the last twenty years.

4. Is it plausible that Roland Gallo would arrange to have Buck Fister killed after finding out that Buck was responsible for Jill's short career as a call girl? Does Roland prize Jill for what he thinks she is (an independent career woman with no romantic involvements) or for what she truly is (a highly vulnerable woman with a desperate need for security)?

5. Are Fiona and Jill drawn sympathetically? Does the reader feel a camaraderie with them or are they merely catalysts for the action around them?

6. What is Noel's attraction to Sage? Is it merely to get to her sister, or is there an emotional attachment between them?

7. Liza feels that her children are keeping her from a writing career. Even today, women feel that they must make choices between career and children. Contrast the two eras. Is it possible for women to "have it all?"

8. Does Portia's discovery of her lesbianism seem at odds with her conventional upbringing? Does environment influence sexuality and our sexual choices, or is it an innate trait, something we are born with?

9. Although Jill vows her prostitution is a "game," the consequences are deadly serious for her and those around her. Is it likely that a woman today would sleep with men for money even if she did not need the money? Is it a thrillseeking mechanism?

10. At one point, Sage makes a pass at her stepfather after being spurned by her husband. Discuss the consequences of her actions: is it incest even though they are not related by blood?

11. Only one of Caroline's daughters, Liza, has had children, and that daughter is the one she seems closest to. Is it because of her children that they enjoy this closeness?

12. What is the significance of "Higgsie," the homeless woman who might have, at one time, been a doctor's wife? Is it a warning not to get swallowed up in a husband's identity, or an alarm to say, "this can happen to you?"

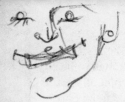

Nelson District C.U. - Vernon

337071

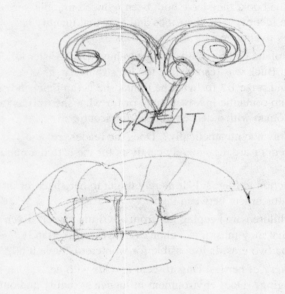

GREAT

but also in bile, blood, brain tissue, milk, nerve fibers, liver, and kidneys . . . to mention just a few.

Cholesterol plays a large part in the formation of gallstones and is seen in hardening of the arteries. It also is found in tuberculosis cysts and in cancerous tissues. I'd say that cholesterol really gets around. Those who blame cholesterol troubles on eating eggs more often than two or three times weekly should look around some more.

Now that we are on the subject of cholesterol, let's take a slower, impartial look. First, let me list a few factual combinations regarding blood-serum cholesterol levels:

1. There are a lot of persons with a high cholesterol level who do not include fat in their daily diet.
2. There are a lot of persons who have a low or normal cholesterol level who do include fat in their daily diet.
3. More fat people have higher cholesterol levels than the normally non-fat people.
4. Many fat people with high cholesterol levels, who lose weight on low calorie, fat-free diets still have high cholesterol levels.

This might be likened to the diabetic who spills over his sugar in his urine, and then, upon greatly reducing his sugar intake, still sees no change in the sugar spill in the urine. The problem lies NOT in the intake of sugar, but rather in the abnormal metabolic utilization of the sugar. Many diabetics have been found to have an antibody formation which is actually resistant to their own insulin. Since we're on the subject, it's a good idea to remember that the diabetic usually has his own insulin in his pancreas but the amount that is eventually available for use is inadequate.

Sounds familiar, like the antibody interference with the "sparking substance" from the thyroid, doesn't it?

We have had patients with high cholesterol levels along with high blood fat levels (hyperlipidemia), who were on fat-free diets along with restricted caloric intake. Yet, their abnormal levels were not affected by weight loss through diet alone. However, these same patients, when given the Supplement, along with liberal proteins, even with some fat, with no refined sugars and starches, promptly began to drop to normal levels. Certain conclusions can and should be drawn from this. And now let's conclude our definitions.

CALORIE: Here, I believe, is a grossly misinterpreted word. By reducing the unit intake, you are reducing the potential amount of energy available to you in its source. While proteins have caloric value, they should not be considered as purely fuel, but more importantly, as a vital and necessary *repair material for all living tissue.*

To review:

The two fuels are carbohydrates and fats. The carbohydrates are normally a quick source of energy and heat. However, too many of the refined or commercial sugars (carbohydrates) are commonly used by potentially overweight people so that the glycogen stored up as available fuel is unused . . . finally converting to fat tissue. By discontinuing the intake of these unnecessary carbohydrates, the glycogen storage will cease and no more excess body fat will accumulate. It follows then, that so long as the body fat remains as the sole fuel available, only it will be burned. In terms of potential energy available, the fuel with the most calorie value would be the one fuel to use and, very clearly, this describes the superiority of fat as that fuel.

Here is a partial list of the human tissues derived from protein:

Hair	Nerves
Skin	Blood Vessels
Nails	Lymph Vessels
Muscles	Brain
Glands	

This should give you a pretty clear insight into the importance of protein. Restricted calorie diets just cannot provide enough protein to keep all of these vital tissues functioning at top efficiency. The wear and tear process of functioning, living tissue must be equaled by the constant re-supply of adequate protein. There are NO substitutes. Once again I must caution you: the amount of protein eaten should be no more than the body can successfully use up.

CHAPTER II

A Guide to Eating

WHAT NOT TO EAT OR DRINK

BEFORE you can lose weight, you must stop gaining. In order to stop gaining it is necessary to know the source of the weight gain. Why one gains is something else again. Earlier in this book I stated that I don't just put people on diets without first giving them some understanding of the overall problem affecting them. I don't expect them to become nutritional experts, but I do expect them to eventually stand on their own feet. I can do no less for you . . . the readers of this book.

There's an old saying: "He who does not mind his belly . . . will hardly mind anything else." Let me assume that you do mind your belly, else why would you have bought this book? However, minding the belly or just nonchalantly declaring, "I'm going on a diet" isn't enough either. The first chapter should already have enlightened you as to why you can gain, while others cannot and do not. You have also been introduced to the food group known as carbohydrates. The next step is to familiarize yourself with the various foods or items making up this group. I'm sure that you are no stranger to them.

Forget the calories for the present. They are units . . . nothing else, and no one ever became fat from units. It is the carbohydrates, which have a potential energy value measured in calories or units, that can and do convert to fat.

Heading the list are the products *containing or made from the refined sugars*. These are the usual commercial sugars and not to be confused with the *natural sugars* found in *fruits* and certain vegetables. Natural vitamins and minerals are also found in many of these. Yet the same vitamins and minerals have to be added in synthetic form to the various refined or commercial products. Because of this artificiality, I would urge you to be well advised about the sales exhortations emphasizing the virtues of enriched or fortified products. They may sound impressive . . . nothing more. But let's get on with it . . . and name names.

THE PASTRIES:

Here are the dough products (already a carbohydrate), but with commercial sugar generously added. Such tasty but useless empty items as *pies;* regardless of being "mother's" "home baked" or "bakery baked," pie is pie and out.

This also includes all *cakes, cookies, doughnuts* (sugared or not) . . . just say *all pastries*.

THE ROUTINE
DOUGH PRODUCTS:

Bread . . . no matter if dark, light, "diet bread" (good for a sickly laugh) . . . no matter if thin sliced or thick sliced. As long as bread is baked from dough . . . it's bread.

Then, the other dough products
. . . *rolls, biscuits, crackers, bread
sticks.*

*Pasta . . . spaghetti, macaroni,
noodles* and similar dough products.

Cereals . . . frosted or not frosted
. . . despite the "enrichment"
with iron-ore, vitamins, or the
beefed-up protein. They are still
mainly 75 to 80 or more percent
carbohydrate.

MORE GOODIES:

Ice cream, candies, all *sugar-
sweetened drinks. Jellies, jams,
preserves, rice, potatoes, corn,
dried beans, lima beans, beets,
parsnips* (peas and carrots are
moderately carbohydrate). *Yoghurt* (the flavored ones with the
sugar-sweetened goo at the bottom of the container). Even milk
has lactose (milk sugar) remain-
ing.

THE DRINKS:

Beer. (If you have a weight problem, beer is one of the most fattening drinks of all.) This doesn't
apply to the non-gainers who
drink beer . . . more power to
them.

*Cocktails, all alcohol drinks, li-
queurs, sweet wines.* Beer . . .
beer. (Forget the "happy drinkers" in the TV commercials.
They are models. Go to the tav-
erns to see the real thing.)

SANDWICHES:

What is in the sandwich is usually not fattening (except for the jelly sandwich), but it's the *two slices of bread*. Stop using the bread as a vehicle to bring the contents to your mouth.

BATTER: You can *fry all you like* (safflower oil or margarine), *but do not dip in batter or eat batter-fried food.* Batter is usually flour or meal or bread crumbs or cracker crumbs. These are carbohydrates.

SOUPS: Avoid *thickened* soups (flour usually added). Stick to *clear soup* or *consomme.* Vegetable soups usually contain the *wrong vegetables* such as corn, potatoes, beans. The same applies to *chowders.* Creamed soups don't contain cream but flour.

AVOID THESE
FRUITS COMPLETELY: *Apricots, bananas, dates* and all dried fruits or candied fruits. Blue grapes, plums, cherries, pears, apples. Confine yourself mostly to moderate amounts of grapefruit or oranges, tangerines, fresh cranberries or rhubarb (artificially sweetened) and fresh pineapple. Unsweetened juices from the above.

This about covers the everyday carbohydrates. Learn the list. Avoid them if you want to stop gaining and don't want to interfere with losing. Concentrate freely on proteins and green vegetables. Be sure your protein intake is adequate . . . not all at one time. If you need the Supplement . . . it can make a great difference.

WHEN AND WHAT TO EAT

The need for protein is a daily requirement. Without the protein the efficiency of your utilizing apparatus will become impaired. The amount of your protein intake depends upon your individual capacity to fully utilize it.

If you wish to go it without the metabolic supplement, your protein intake must be kept within your individual limits. You will have to find your level by testing varying amounts of daily protein intake. I have found that many individuals, because of a conditioned reluctance to eat too much, actually eat too little protein, resulting in slow or even no progress. Too little can be as much a handicap as too much. Yet, with the prescribed Supplement, you have a much greater freedom in how much protein you can eat.

The daily purpose remains constant. This is to activate the available excess body fat as fuel, or your sole source of energy. The amount of protein intake must be that which you can fully utilize. The suggested regimen below will help you to determine this.

BREAKFAST
Start with a hamburger plus egg or eggs
(cooked any way you like)
or
Steak (5 or 6 oz.) with eggs
or
Bacon (3-4 strips) with eggs
Coffee or tea (artificially sweetened)

If you would like ½ grapefruit or some unsweetened juice, leave it for later in the day or at night. If you want some lunch, try some cottage cheese with salad vegetables or some sardines, tuna, or salmon. (Drain off the oil.)

DINNER

Steak, hamburger meat, roast, chicken.
Turkey, fish (if fried, not in batter).
Cooked green vegetables (regular serving of spinach, asparagus, string beans, mushrooms, broccoli, etc.).

Coffee or tea (no milk), artificially sweetened.

This can be a test for you. If you are not more than a few pounds overweight, and you still do not lose, your portions of protein may be too much for you. Try eliminating lunch or reducing the portions of meat.

Remember this: even if you do lose weight without the Supplement, you still are NOT doing anything to affect or influence your own individual metabolic limitation. People do lose weight on other diets, mainly because they are eating small portions (restricted calories). Yet it is unlikely that they can or will continue on such limited food intake for a prolonged period of time.

The excellent results with the participating members of the Boston Police must be attributed, in my opinion, to the fact that all have been, and still are, taking the Supplement. Most persons are now more interested in the long range results, rather than in the immediate loss of some weight because of restricted total food intake. They realize that eventually you have to discontinue inadequate portions to maintain functional efficiency.

It may sound strange, but in many instances I have to urge some of the BPD members, as well as private patients, to eat more protein. With the Supplement it is quite common to find the best losers among the best eaters of meat. New patients frequently have been so completely oriented to restricted calories (or just not eating) that they are very hesitant to eat as much protein as I constantly urge them to. Look at it this way . . . the more excess fat available to be ignited and used, the more protein required to replace the cast-off tissue cells and prevent lessening the efficiency of the metabolic apparatus.

If you can find your own level through just limiting your protein intake . . . and lose weight . . . fine. If you cannot seem to lose and find restricted food intake depressing, then I would advise that you seek the aid and cooperation of your physician, who would be able to prescribe the small doses of the Supplement. I am strongly opposed to the use of the appetite suppressors. I believe them to be potentially dangerous for many unwary dieters. I am not trying to cut down your appetite. I want you to eat, but eat protein . . . not carbohydrate. Those appetite pills, assuming that they did cause you to eat much less, have no selective action. They (or any type of medication), can't stop you from eating only carbohydrates or create a preference for protein. Your ultimate goal is to instinctively select protein and to reject carbohydrates (the useless ones . . . not the natural ones in fruit and vegetables). Pies, cakes, cookies, doughnuts, ice cream, candies, sweet drinks, beer, booze, pasta, and the fortified breakfast cereals contribute nothing essential to your health or well-being. You could very well live without them. But you cannot live without protein.

A DIVERSIFIED LIST OF PROTEINS

There is no lack of variety when choosing from the available proteins. You need not go hungry . . . even if you miss having bread or rolls. Some of the following are always available. And remember: you can fry in butter, or margarine, or oil if you wish, but do not dip in batter, which is carbohydrate (flour, meal, bread crumbs, etc.).

STEAKS
HAMBURGERS (no rolls, of
(course)
ROAST BEEF
LAMB CHOPS
ROAST LAMB
ROAST PORK
PORK CHOPS
VEAL
CHICKEN
TURKEY
DUCK and GOOSE
BACON
HAM
SAUSAGES
COLD MEATS (beef, lamb,
chicken, turkey, freely)
PREPARED MEATS (in limited
amounts because they con-
tain other ingredients)

LOBSTERS (can be dipped in
melted butter, but avoid
sweet dressing in baked
lobster)
SHRIMP (cocktail, fried, no
batter)
CLAMS (cocktail, fried, no
batter)
ALL FRESH FISH (cook any
style, except no batter)
SARDINES, SALMON, TUNA
(with oil drained)

Here are some acceptable combinations:

STEAK and EGGS
HAMBURGER and EGGS
BACON and EGGS
HAM and EGGS
SAUSAGES and EGGS

There is a vast difference between protein and protein-containing food products. Meat, fish, and fowl are mainly protein with
varying amounts of fat.

Prepared meats or the sandwich meats may be labeled as
containing "all beef," yet actually this only means that pork or
any other type of meat was not included in the making of the
product. The label does NOT read "all meat" since there can

be, and usually are, non-meat ingredients added. Many contain some cereal, corn syrup and other carbohydrates mixed in with the beef. Obviously, because of this, the label cannot read "all meat." It merely identifies the kind of meat used. Unfortunately, the amount of meat protein is much less than that found in all meat products.

Now perhaps you understand why I recommend eating freely of steak, chicken, hamburger, fish, etc. and also why I discourage more than a limited intake of the prepared meats. Always bear in mind this fact: you did not become fat merely because you ate carbohydrates. It's because you ate carbohydrates too much and too often. Sadly, what's too much for you isn't too much for many others.

DAIRY PRODUCTS

This is a protein-containing group. It must be understood correctly. Non-fat milk, even though the fat has been removed, still has carbohydrate (lactose or milk-sugar), despite the removal of half the original calories. If you drank enough non-fat milk, the volume of lactose carbohydrate could be fattening . . . even with reduced total calories. *Both non-fat and whole milk should be restricted during the early stages of the weight reducing program.* You can use some to "lighten" your coffee if you don't like it black. You can even use some heavy cream, but in limited amounts. We'd rather have those fat calories in more protein.

Many persons refer to themselves as "health nuts." What a quaint expression. I don't really know what a "health nut" is, but if eating yoghurt and other self-styled "health foods" is the ingredient for a special type of health, then perhaps the "health nut" is well-named. There are no mystical, super-health or reducing powers in yoghurt or any other fermented milk products. The protein content is the same as in any milk product. There is also the same amount of carbohydrate as in any milk products. Making yoghurt from non-fat milk merely removes the fat, thus reducing the calorie value by half. But it still is no less fattening. The carbohydrate is still there. It amuses me (painfully) to see the innocents going on a yoghurt kick eagerly selecting the temptingly flavored little packages modestly labeled with such tastebud-teasing names as prune whip, strawberry, vanilla, and pineapple. Sadly I watch the poor neglected plain yoghurt being rudely cast aside while eager hands pulled at the flavored cousins. I can almost hear the poor plain yoghurt sadly saying, "Don't they know that the enticing flavor is a blob of sugary, preserve-like goo at the bottom of the little package? How can they miss it when they have to stir the whole mixture?" It's much like pouring yourself a glass of non-fat milk, then adding several tablespoons of some flavored marmalade or preserve. Would you do that if you were on any type of reducing diet? If you must have yoghurt . . . at least pick only the plain.

Cheese is a multi-variety food. Cottage cheese has less volume than does processed hard cheese. Creamed cottage cheese doesn't vary much from the non-fat or skimmed milk type. Both are mostly water . . . about 78 to 80%. Both have about four to five grams of protein per ounce . . . approximately one gram of carbohydrate for each . . . and a total energy value of about thirty calories per ounce in the creamed and about twenty-five calories per ounce in the non-fat type. The few extra calories result from the cream added.

Thus, while no one really becomes fat from cottage cheese, it isn't an ideal source of protein. It makes a good filler, but doesn't and shouldn't replace meat as a vital source of protein.

In hard cheese (American, Cheddar, etc.), one ounce has about 35 to 40% water. The energy value is divided as protein and fat. There are approximately 7 grams of protein and about 9 grams of fat. The total calorie value per ounce is approximately 110 to 120. Make this comparison for yourself: one ounce of cottage cheese would have an energy potential of about 25 to 30 calories, while one ounce of Cheddar or American would have a potential of about 110 to 120 calories. Yet, I wouldn't push hard cheese to any great extent since about 4 ounces would have an energy value of about 440 to 480 calories with the bulk of the calories coming from the fat . . . not the protein. I'd prefer the same or more calories from a like amount of meat.

I'm not against fat in the diet, but certain conditions must be observed. As long as you have plenty of excess fat to be made available as fuel, you should NOT add very much from the outside. Let's concentrate most of the calorie intake in protein.

A GENERAL GUIDE FOR CHOOSING FOODS

Here is how to simplify the whole procedure. Whenever you consider any food item always ask yourself: Is it carbohydrate or does it contain any carbohydrate? This is your key to avoiding the potentially fattening foods.

It's not how many calories are listed, but rather *what is the source of the calories*. The calories are not the fattening factor. They only determine the potential nutritional or energy value of the particular food item.

Listening to the various food commercials will provide good examples of how to misinterpret the significance of the calorie. For example, in one commercial a young woman is almost bubbling over with "directed" enthusiasm as she extolls the virtues of her diet drink. She announces, "This is a *real* diet drink." Why? Simply because it contains only two calories per portion. Then, as an afterthought she adds, "and it's also *sugar-free.*" The sugar-free statement should have been made first. This is the core of the matter. It is the sugar-free element which maks this drink authentically non-fattening. The fact about the two calories merely qualifies the drink as having little or no nutritional value. To prove a point, I could take this same drink, convert it into a high calorie drink by adding some safflower oil or some protein extract. Yet so long as no sugar was added, it would still be a non-fattening drink. Of course, I won't vouch for its taste, but the point will be proved.

I would urge you to always read the ingredients listed on the label when you are assessing the potential of any food product. If there is carbohydrate (sugar or starch) listed, try to determine how much of the total calorie content is made up by the carbohydrates. The label may emphasize the diet value of the product by stressing the low calories, but this does not and cannot hide the carbohydrate content.

Here is a good example. Fats, as a specific food group, has the highest calorie value of the three food groups. *But fats are not fattening.* Because they have more than double the amount of calories found in the other two groups, *fats represent the greatest source of potential energy and heat.*

Understand though, I am NOT urging you to go all out on fats because of this. Why should you when you already have a generous supply of fat piled up on your body? That's the fuel we want you to use for your energy, while burning off the excess amount.

The BPD Program doesn't restrict fats, per se. If you like some fat on your meat, or from other sources . . . help yourself. Enjoy! I happen to like eggs, with bacon, steak, hamburgers, or, many times . . . just eggs. Of course, this information isn't going to please the cholesterol alarmists who are constantly urging all abstinence from fat. I'd like to clear up some confusion about this matter. While fats may contain cholesterol, they do not *make* cholesterol. *The body makes cholesterol.* Many of your tissues contain cholesterol normally. There are many individuals with high cholesterol blood levels who do not have any fat in their daily diets. Likewise, there are many individuals with low or normal levels who do eat fats freely in their diets. There are many heart attack victims who were on fat-free diets for years.

There are many heart attack victims who had normal cholesterol levels. You can formulate many combinations, but one fact remains constant. Eating fats, per se, no more causes high cholesterol levels in certain individuals than does eating sugar cause diabetes in other individuals. Let's face up to the hard fact. A metabolic disorder of hereditary origin is involved and dietary changes alone are not going to have any direct affect upon this disorder. This leads us directly to the Supplement. While it does not affect the hereditary fact, it does supply some corrective additions to an existing deficiency. Remember, the thyroid gland itself is doing its job. What happens to the "sparking substance" after it leaves the gland is the key to the metabolic disorder.

The addition of the Supplement has made a great difference in functional end results. For example, I have checked considerable numbers of patients for cholesterol and blood fat contents, comparing those who were on the Supplement with those who were not. The results clearly showed the overwhelming advantage of the Supplement in keeping the cholesterol and blood lipids within normal limits. If you are not taking the Supplement, then naturally I cannot expect to find the same response to fats, etc. as those who are. In short, I would NOT recommend a free intake of fats unless you were taking something to affect the hereditary metabolic defect. This is the function and reason for the Supplement.

I happen to like eggs . . . and some fat on meat. I eat an average of four eggs daily. I like hard-boiled eggs at night . . . sort of a late snack. But remember that I have been taking the Supplement for more than twenty-five years. Your eating habits will have to be influenced by whether or not you are taking the Supplement. It's as simple as that.

A Specific Meal Guide

BREAKFAST

Steak and eggs, hamburgers and eggs, bacon and eggs, ham and eggs, kippers (or any kind of fish) and eggs.
Scrambled eggs and cottage cheese (not a lot of protein).
Salami or bologna (not the best source of protein) and eggs.
Cold roast or chicken (there is no law that says you can't eat this for breakfast).
Tomato or grapefruit juice (unsweetened).
Half grapefruit or fresh strawberries (no sugar added). You can even add a little cream, but no non-dairy creams.

LUNCH

Green salad. (You do not need much protein if your breakfast contained a large amount of meat)
Hard boiled eggs . . . sardines . . . tuna
NO sandwiches

DINNER

Soup. Clear soup, bouillon, consommé. (Be sure soup isn't flour thickened.)
Have a generous portion of meat, fowl or fish. (You should now be ready for more protein.)
Cooked green vegetables (see detailed list).
Green salad. (any non-sugar sweetened dressing).
Cranberries or rhubarb (artificially sweetened).
Coffee, tea, sugar-free drinks.

The size of your portion will depend upon whether or not you are taking the Supplement.

You can forgo milk for the present. Nothing drastic will happen. (I never touch the stuff.)

Use your own judgment: if you like fresh cranberries or rhubarb, get the fresh products and sweeten with saccharin. Beware of the so-called "diet products." Too many are called that because they have not added sugar. However, they still contain their natural sugar.

As the ancient Greek philosopher Socrates said, "Beware of those foods that tempt you to eat when you are not hungry, and of those liquors that tempt you to drink when you are not thirsty." I believe the sly old philosopher knew much about the tempting sweets even then, not to mention the non-water drinks. His point is well taken.

Here are some vegetables and fruits you *can* eat. They contain natural vitamin C and other important "musts."

ASPARAGUS
BRUSSELS SPROUTS
BROCCOLI
CABBAGE
CAULIFLOWER
CELERY
CHICORY
CUCUMBERS
ESCAROLE
EGGPLANT
LETTUCE
MUSHROOMS
OKRA
SCALLIONS
GREEN PEPPERS
RADISHES
SAUERKRAUT (not with sugar
    added)

SQUASH (summer)
STRING BEANS
TOMATOES
TURNIPS
WATERCRESS
CANTALOUPE
GRAPEFRUIT
GRAPEFRUIT JUICE (unsweet-
    ened)
ORANGE
ORANGE JUICE (unsweet-)
    ened)
STRAWBERRIES (fresh, arti-
    ficially sweetened)
TANGERINES
(The fruits listed are lowest
    in carbohydrates and rich-
    est in vitamin C.)

SOME FREQUENTLY ASKED QUESTIONS

1. *Can you eat boiled or broiled lobsters dipped in butter or margarine?*
   Yes. The meat of lobster is practically ALL protein. However, be wary of the dressing or stuffing with baked lobster. It is usually sweetened and contains crumbs (carbohydrate). You can also dip in cocktail sauce . . . providing it has no sugar. Try shrimps fried in butter or safflower margarine. Don't dip in batter.

2. *Must everything be broiled or boiled?*
   Of course not. You can fry freely in safflower oil, margarine, or butter. But . . . no dipping in batter. Try dipping in beaten egg. There's NO carbohydrate in eggs.

3. *Must you have only the white meat of chicken? What about skin?*
   Eat any part of the chicken you like. This also applies to turkey. Try duck and goose . . . if you like. The skin is protein, but most of the conventional calorie restricting diets outlaw the skin because of the fat underneath which adds calories. Remember, the calories aren't fattening . . . only the carbohydrates are.

4. *Can you have whipped cream?*
   Yes. Cream is all fat, whipped or unwhipped, until you add any sugar for sweetening. Use artificial sweetener. There will still be *no sugar* in cream.

5. *What about condiments?*
   No one ever became fat from mustard, ketchup (beware of some sugar in it) pepper, and spices. If you seem to retain fluid, then you may have to restrict your salt intake. (Fluid retention is NOT caused by salt, but is frequently associated with obesity and defective metabolic function.) The addition

of the Supplement has aided many overweights with fluid problems.

6. *What about salmon . . . sardines . . . tuna?*
   Eat them . . . they're fish. You don't have to look for water packed cans. Just drain off the added oil. The natural oil is in the fish. You do not need the added calories from the non-natural oil. Eat enough, since a can of sardines containing 4 or 5 small fish doesn't add up to much protein. Salmon is excellent. It is precooked; thus the bones are easily digested and provide good calcium plus other important elements.

7. *What about "social drinking"? Are there any preferred, less-fattening drinks?*
   One drink never made anyone fat, no more than did one piece of candy. It's how often the one drink is repeated in a given period of time. One drink, occasionally, may not be significant. However, for some persons with a weight problem, one drink daily can contribute to unhappy results. Naturally, it would be much better if you didn't drink, but at least let me make some suggestions. For the overweight who identifies beer as one of his frequent and steady pleasures . . . there is NO compromise. Out . . . beer . . . out. Beer is one of the *most fattening* of fatteners for those who have a true obesity problem. I consider it worse than drinking highballs. Cocktails, if not sweetened, are somewhat less "evil" than syrup-sweetened, soft drinks. If you drink at all, at least "nurse" your drink, avoid "freshening" it or having refills. As to wines, sweet wines are *out.* Try to stick to *dry* wines (champagne, etc.).

The over-cocktails business meetings or "happy hours" or the usual pre-dinner drink may have become a way of life or a daily routine for you, but if you are concerned with a weight problem, this routine will have to be changed.

Frequently, I hear the excuses for straying from the charted path. (I must devote a chapter to "My Treasury of Patients' Alibis.") It is so easy to blame various occasions for your own lack of judgment in choosing the right foods. Don't blame it on the wedding, graduation, anniversary, bar-mitzvah, wake, vacation, or any other get-together. You can always find something right to eat or drink. I don't particularly enjoy preaching to you, but someone has to remind you that you do not become fat from vespers or prayers.

Learn to start your day with enough protein to activate your supply of excess body fat. Draw your energy requirements from the burning fat. You don't have to re-supply protein again at noon if your morning intake is sufficient. Your fuel ("body fat") is still there in a constant but gradually diminishing supply. Your evening meal should then re-supply enough protein to keep the burning apparatus active for more hours. If you are NOT taking the Supplement, you may have to search for your adequate individual protein level. If you begin to lose, don't be reluctant to eat. If you are not losing sufficiently, your protein intake may have to be somewhat reduced. *Don't restrict your freedom of action by counting calories.* You will either eat more protein or less protein, depending upon your progress. For example, if eight ounces of meat is too much, reduce it to six ounces. Don't reduce the portions too much. Your intake should be enough to activate the burning apparatus. If you lose satisfactorily only by virtually starving yourself, don't rely on this way as the only way. You probably will get better and quicker results if your physician prescribes the Supplement in small doses. You'll also be able to eat larger portions of protein, remember. (The meat eaters among my group are always the best losers.)

A final bit of advice: limit your intake of cold or prepared meats. They contain additives such as cereal, corn syrup, or meal. This applies to the general family of "sandwich meats" . . . bologna, salami, pressed meats. Concentrate on the whole meat products. Beef, lamb, veal, pork.

YOU DON'T HAVE TO BE A HERMIT

Are you afraid to go to parties, dinners, and other social events because you feel that you can't eat anything or that you will go off your diet?

Well, I wouldn't blame you, if you were one of the conventional dieters, armed with your trusty calorie counters, who had to weigh or size-up each morsel of food. I know how easy it is for some other guest or the hostess to coax you to "forget your diet this time." No one surrounded by a group of drinkers and eaters likes to say (unconvincingly), "Everything looks so good . . . but I must watch my diet." How many times have you gone "off watch" with only the slightest coaxing?

Things are going to be different now. You can go to as many affairs as you wish and leave your calorie-counter at home. Better still, throw it away if its presence bothers you. From now on you are going to be following a different philosophy. Your major concern will be: "Is this fattening" or "is there any sugar or other carbohydrate in this particular item?" This means you can forget the calorie counter, but it also means that you must do your homework well and be able to recognize proteins from carbohydrates without constantly referring to a book. Sooner or later you'll be able to adjust the portions to your individual capacity for igniting and utilizing.

Always keep in mind this operational condition: your freedom in portion sizes will depend on whether you are or are not taking the Supplement. If you, with your physician, have found the Supplement vital to your progress, then, in general, you don't have to be concerned with how much you eat. Your concern will be what you eat. You're not being given free rein to just gorge yourself. But if you feel that you did "go overboard," don't fall back on the "I just hate myself" torture line. Learn to compensate for the overloading by skipping calorie volume for a meal or two. This is not saying "don't eat for several days." Your need for protein is constant, but reduce the amount and fill up with more bulky, low-calorie food such as salads, cooked green vegetables, cottage cheese, hard-boiled eggs, etc. Don't eliminate the protein! You always need some to keep the apparatus functioning, and don't have any carbohydrate at the next party or meal.

We are dividing our Program into two phases . . . each with its specific goal. The first phase is concerned mainly with losing the unwanted excess body fat. The second phase, of equal or even greater importance, is concerned with keeping it off permanently. The operations are different because the goals are different. While protein is always vital in either phase, the fuels become interchangeable. For example, in the first phase, it is the excess body fat that must be gotten rid of. Thus, it is the main fuel to burn. Any carbohydrate intake can only detract from the exclusiveness of the fat as the only fuel available. Even a relatively moderate intake of fat from the outside won't, as a rule, interfere with the burning body fat. In fact, it can actually accelerate the combustion.

Conditions are different in phase two. Energy requirements are still constant for you as long as you are alive. But now the fuels that are available as the source for the energy are different in terms of being automatically handy. During phase one, the excess body fat was available. But now that the excess fat is gone (and you should retain the normal fat for its normal functions) fuel must be supplied from the outside. You can either include a sufficient amount of fat such as meat, dairy, fowl, or vegetable fatty oils along with the protein, or you can begin to include small amounts of carbohydrates in the daily fare.

Certain carbohydrates are still a quick source of energy and are useful as a quick fuel . . . and a source of certain vitamins. This refers to the natural carbohydrates found mainly in fresh fruit and vegetables. This still does not apply to the usual commercial or refined sugar products. They were the "varmints" that produced the fat you're trying to get rid of . . . or have already. If you do go back to them; just keep in mind the governing condition for you. If your intake of these particular carbohydrates is too much . . . too often, you are going to be in trouble again. Where you formerly ate a good sized portion of pie or cake, make it half the amount from now on and do not make them a daily habit. This should apply to all desserts.

I mentioned that you don't have to be a hermit even during the first phase; follow this brief guide for party snacks. And remember, no pill in the world will do your picking for you. Selectivity is your responsibility.

HORS D'OEUVRES:	Usually what's on the cracker or piece of toast is essentially non-fattening. You can enjoy the smoked salmon, egg salad, anchovies, caviar, cold meat, sardines. Just leave the cracker or toast.
PLATTERS:	Cocktail franks, meat balls, cheese, cold or hot turkey, sliced chicken, ham, ribs, salmon or tuna salad. Avoid the dough products . . . batters, rolls, etc.
SALADS:	Enjoy mixed fresh salads, sliced tomatoes, cucumbers, radishes, celery, pickles, or even a few olives.
DRINKS:	Sugar-free soft drinks are not usually available at most social events. But don't use this as an excuse to drink the regular sugar-sweetened ones. If you feel that you must have a drink in your hand, have a small jigger of whiskey, well diluted with water or soda. You can sip it slowly or use it to stall

DESSERTS:
the frequent freshenings of the solicitous hostess.
Stay away from sweet wines and beer.
If there are small chunks of fresh fruit
. . . good enough. Let the multi-layered cakes and eclairs ambush some other soul. But if you do stray . . . compensate later.

HOLIDAYS ARE GREAT DAYS ON THE B.P.D. PROGRAM

I used to hear one particular excuse during certain holidays each year. (Other excuses were used for other times.) Anyhow, it seemed to establish a sort of pattern always before the "stepping on the scale" ritual. It always went like this: "You know it was a holiday, doctor, and I just couldn't help myself." Of course it was a holiday. I'm not in some sort of isolation. Still, in my usual kindly manner I would sweetly say: "Ah, you're trying to tell me something . . . something like "I just *had* to go off my diet since there was this man with a gun at my head threatening me if I didn't eat that horrid tempting plate of candied yams and tasteless stuffing with the turkey." I tearfully asked about the other forced "nauseating" items such as rolls, pumpkin pie, or in extreme cases . . . even raisin pie and its cousin, mince pie. In my grief I scarcely dared to ask about the final blow . . . submitting to the indignity of managing some ice cream or having to chew and swallow candy mints (involuntarily, of course).

Strange. Even I used to admire certain ingenious alibis, yet not once did I see any sympathetic response from my scale. My sympathies were extended to those who tried to follow the conventional diets . . . holiday or not. Now I am no longer tearful, but merely display menus for any holiday.

Here are some possibilities for a Thanksgiving menu. (Try
suffering through this diet.)

Tomato or grapefruit juice (unsweetened)
Celery sticks, radishes, olives, scallions
Clear soup, bouillon, consomme
Shrimp cocktail, crabmeat cocktail, fresh fruit cup

Antipasto

Roast turkey (without stuffing), roast chicken, roast beef, leg
   of lamb

Fish (broiled, baked, or fried but not dipped in batter)
Lobster (boiled or broiled, avoid baked lobster because of
   stuffing)

Vegetables (see list on separate page)

Tossed green salad with dressing
Sauerkraut, pickles, pickled tomatoes

Fresh cranberries, rhubarb (artificially sweetened)
Gelatin (artificially sweetened)

Coffee, tea, dry wine, champagne

A SELECTION OF NON-FATTENING RECIPES

SHRIMP REMOULADE
   ¼ cup safflower oil
   2 tablespoons of vinegar
   1 teaspoon paprika
   ½ teaspoon salt
   2 tablespoons prepared hot mustard
   1 tablespoon horseradish
   2 tablespoons green scallion tops
      Stir well, then add ½ to ¾ lbs. cooked shrimps. Toss
      well, then chill.

TUNA SALAD
> Tuna
> Chopped onions
> Green peppers
> Chopped celery
> Tomatoes (small cut)
> Add some mayonnaise and some lemon juice to taste.

BAKED HALIBUT
> Coat baking dish with safflower oil, margarine, or butter. Add salt and pepper to taste.
> Sprinkle with paprika and parsley.
> Pour ½ to ¼ cup of cream over fish.
> Bake until done.

BAKED HADDOCK
> Coat baking dish as above. Add sliced onions and sliced green peppers. Salt moderately. Pour can of tomato soup (undiluted) over fish. Top with pieces of butter or safflower oil margarine. Bake for about an hour.

SHRIMP SALAD
> Cooked shrimps
> Hard boiled eggs
> Diced celery
> Place on bed of lettuce leaves.
> Serve with mayonnaise and lemon wedges.

CHICKEN SALAD (BPD Special)
> Cut large amounts of chicken, tongue and swiss cheese into long strips. Pour avocado dressing over. Place on a bed of lettuce. Serves 8.

AVOCADO DRESSING
> 1 peeled, mashed avocado
> Combine with ⅓ cup lemon juice, 2 tablespoons vinegar, ¼ cup safflower oil, a pinch of dry mustard, a dash of Worcestershire sauce and salt to taste. Beat well with eggbeater.

CUCUMBERS IN SOUR CREAM
  Slice cucumbers and onions thinly.
  Add vinegar (artificially sweetened) and sour cream.
  Salt and pepper to taste. Keep refrigerated.

MARINATED STEAK
  Mix ⅓ cup safflower oil, 2 tablespoons lemon juice,
  garlic and parsley minced. Marinate steak in mixture
  for 3 hours, turning often. Drain well. Broil steak,
  adding safflower oil, margarine or butter, if you wish.

HAMBURGER IN TOMATO SAUCE
  (A favorite of mine)
  Mix some diced green peppers with crumbled hamburger meat. Fry slowly in safflower oil or meat's own
  fat. Drain off fatty liquid. Add a can of tomato puree
  (or two cans) plus a can of mushrooms. Simmer for
  10 to 15 minutes.

BROCCOLI PARMESAN
  Boil broccoli slowly in salted water until barely tender.
  Place butter or safflower oil margarine in saucepan and
  sprinkle with garlic salt. Saute broccoli in mixture.
  Cover with grated Parmesan cheese and bake in oven
  until brown.

FRENCH FRIED TURNIPS
  Peel turnips. Cut into French fry strips. Fry in safflower oil until brown, turning often. Add salt, if you
  wish.

FROSTED HOT ASPARAGUS
  Cook asparagus until tender. Drain. Beat some egg
  whites until fluffy. Fold in some mayonnaise. Frost the
  mixture thoroughly. Place under broiler until light
  brown.

GREEN BEANS, ITALIAN STYLE
  Heat 4 tablespoons of safflower oil. Saute a cup of

chopped onions, a bay leaf, clove, garlic, and salt to taste for about 5 minutes. Add a can or two each of tomatoes and green beans. Cook slowly for about 30 minutes.

There are no carbohydrates in these recipes. However, because of the fats, there are plenty of calories. So if you are taking the Supplement, eat freely. If not, keep your portions limited.

"BOVINE HASH"
Cut leftover cold roast beef into bite size chunks. Dice some onions. Add some chopped hard boiled eggs. Add enough safflower margarine or butter to moisten the mix. Serve this with a salad.

ANTIPASTO A LA APPETITE
Cover a large platter with lettuce leaves. Place the contents of a can of tuna (drained) over the lettuce.
Surround with slices of salami, small squares of Cheddar cheese, olives, and a generous sprinkling of pimento. Pour a little safflower oil and vinegar over to suit individual taste.

CUCUMBER SALAD
Dissolve one package lime gelatin (artificially sweetened) in hot water. Add vinegar and cool. Add teaspoon onion juice (or finely minced onion), 1 cup sour cream and 1 cup mayonnaise. Add 2 cups chopped cucumbers. Pour mixture into molds. Cool. Makes dozen or more molds.

SOUR CREAM DRESSING
Mix well:
½ cup sour cream
½ cup mayonnaise
1 tablespoon horseradish
and chopped onion

BLEU CHEESE DRESSING
    Mix well:
¾ cup safflower oil
¼ cup vinegar
¼ cup paprika
    add
    Crumbled bleu cheese
1 teaspoon lemon juice
½ cup mayonnaise
1 tablespoon dry mustard
1 tablespoon Worcestershire sauce
    Blend well and refrigerate for several hours. Serve at room temperature.

HOLLANDAISE SAUCE
    Blend:
    3 egg yolks and 2 tablespoons lemon juice in blender at low speed until smooth. Slowly add ½ cup melted margarine. This can be used on broccoli, asparagus, cauliflower and fish dishes.

APPETIZERS
    Stuff celery with Bleu cheese and sprinkle with paprika.
    Shrimps on toothpicks. Combine ketchup, lemon juice and horseradish for dip.
    Roll slices of salami around dill pickles.

CHOPPED LIVER
    Pan fry chicken livers and onions in safflower margarine. Put through meat grinder. Add hard boiled eggs. Mix together well and mold. Serve on a bed of lettuce.

LITTLE CHUNKS
    Small cubes of cheese, olives, and pickles.

CHAPTER III

Gone . . . But Not Forgotten

HOW TO KEEP IT OFF AFTER YOU'VE LOST IT

MERELY losing weight presents no great problem. That is, of course, if you don't care how you do it. Complete starvation, if followed long enough, is a sure way to lose weight (plus other things along the way). But, even so, how long could you go along with that kind of "diet"? So what did you accomplish? You are compelled to start eating again, following your usual habits, and the lost weight soon says "hello again."

Diets, exercise programs, etc. are useless, and even dangerous, unless you can continue them safely and permanently. So the type of diet you start with can usually be the answer to the question, "What's going to happen later on?" No one can continue indefinitely on a 500 calorie . . . or even a 1,000 calorie diet. How many times have you been advised, when you ask about snacks at night or at other times, to just eat "a few slivers of carrots or some celery?" You might just as well eat some wood shavings for all the good these will do to appease your craving for something. So forget the slivers . . . forget the ever-omnipotent calories . . . and have yourself a ball. Eat some slivers (good-sized ones) of cold roast or cold chicken or even a hard-boiled egg. Just be certain that it's your "friendly protein," NOT the "unfriendly carbohydrate." Of course, you could eat too much of protein also, especially if you are not getting the extra spark from the Supplement. But you still will not accumulate any excess body fat from the protein. The carbohydrates will always claim the credit for that.

Unfortunately, we all too often confuse hunger with boredom. I wonder how many of us really know what true hunger is. Missing a meal or two can scarcely be compared with those unfortunates in other lands who miss meals constantly, and when they do manage to have a meal, it is most inadequate. Those poor souls know what hunger is. It's with them day in and day out . . . never letting up. Our hunger isn't remotely similar.

Some persons think about food or eating simply because they haven't anything more important to occupy them. The restlessness of boredom begins to overtake the stomach senses. For want of something to do, they begin to look for escape routes . . . and eating heads the list. Some find it in smoking . . . others in drinking . . . some even in the extremes of drugs. But face it, most find it in the always convenient, ever-pleasurable escape of food.

Do you need examples? I have pockets full of them. Let's start with a man and wife . . . or any other couple. They have just finished eating a substantial meal . . . six or seven o'clock. Next, they decide to go to a cinema (movie, before the admission prices took wings). At the picture palace they seat themselves on luxuriously uncomfortable seats, following which they extend the head and neck and then stare at the screen. The physical activity involved may even be increased by a few subtle yawns. The inactivity of looking ahead and doing nothing soon gives birth to the first emotions of boredom. The escapism on the screen is not enough. An even better escape is recalled . . . in the lobby. Ah, the popcorn machine, the candy counter, the bubbling fountain of syrupy soft drinks. Succor is at hand. Soon the box or boxes of popcorn are dipped into, after which the mouths become aggressively active. Of course, the sprinkling of salt soon leads to, "I'm thirsty, how about you?" And then sweetened drinks are soon guzzled. Then thoughts return to visions of the candy counter. Well, after all, salt is salt, so a little "sweet" would just be the right finishing touch. Exit . . . to the candy counter . . . for a bar or two.

What's the point of this recitation? Have you forgotten that these citizens had just finished a substantial meal before they arrived at the cinema? Do you think they were actually hungry only an hour or so after that meal? Boredom has many faces. You can sit at home after the evening meal . . . just read or watch television or even listen to the radio. Now, the kindly guardians of our destinies have faithfully provided us with TV snack trays on which you can conveniently place the TV snacks. Watching and munching is NOT hunger. It is pure unadulterated habit or conditioning, which many of us unresistingly accept.

These are some of the "fun habits" you'll have to change. Too bad they don't serve "jerky" or "cold hamburger-on-a-stick" or even a bag of "steak-chunkies" . . . anything but the conventional goodies. Keeping it off is a horse of a different color compared with taking it off. Here's why: once you have burned up the excess body fat, you will no longer have a ready pile of fuel (fat) available for burning. You will now have to supply fuel from the outside as you require the energy. This means either carbohydrates or fats . . . or both. Protein still will be number one . . . regardless. Your need for protein never ceases.

Let's take a "case" as an example.

This person has lost weight by burning up his excess body fat. He now has just the normal body fat available for its normal use. Fuel must now be provided daily from the outside. He could, let's say, rely entirely upon protein, plus some vegetables and some natural vitamin-containing fruit. Yet protein is mainly a tissue builder, not a true fuel. While protein supplies most of the daily food ingested, tissues (muscle) are being built up. There is, however, no longer any excess body fat to melt and get rid of and to offset the weight being gained by the protein tissue building-up process. To put it more plainly, you could be gaining weight . . . not because of excess fat accumulation, but because of extra muscle building up. (This is how an athlete should gain weight, if he wants to. Not by gain due to fat accumulation, but by actually building up more muscle tissue. This, of course, requires protein.)

Back to our example. He doesn't need as much protein as before, so his intake can be reduced. But he still does need fuel, so he can begin adding some carbohydrate to his daily diet. This doesn't mean the useless types such as candy, pies and cakes (unless in small quantities). It does mean, however, some whole grain bread (not as much as he used to eat . . . nor as often), even potato and the formerly forbidden vegetables . . . but, again, in smaller and less frequent amounts.

If you have taken the Supplement during the losing period, and afterwards discontinued it, then your regular limited spark level is back again. This means that the total intake of everything must be kept within that limit. If the Supplement is continued, you don't have to be so limited in portions.

I must remind you of this important fact: What was fattening during your losing period is just as fattening afterward . . . and always will be. Don't think of your future as one of constant dieting. Instead, think of it as a new and better way of nutrition and well-being.

If you go off your eating program on occasion and eat or drink a little too much of the wrong things . . . don't panic or shoot yourself. Just learn to compensate by skipping a meal or two or by adequately reducing portions for a time. It is that simple to make your own adjustments . . . to keep your size constant. *Don't try to keep the scale weight exactly the same every day.* It's well nigh impossible. One can gain a pound or two occasionally, due to temporary fluid retention or other causes. It is not related to any accumulation of excess body fat. If your size begins to go up or clothes really begin to feel tighter, then you don't need a scale to tell you what's happening. I haven't been on a scale for many years. I don't want to know numbers. I am completely satisfied knowing that if I formerly had a 42 inch waistline and now, for quite some time, have a 32 inch waistline (loose), I just can't weigh the same as when the 42 size was king. Let your size changes be the real criterion.

THE STORIES IN THE MAIL

It is not surprising that I have received thousands of letters, since the story of the Boston Police Diet and Weight Control Program has enjoyed widespread and repeated coverage by the national news media. Police activities always seem to interest the public. Now, with the familiar image of the "fat cop" being so favorably altered, the image is all the more interesting.

The letters are sent either to my office (most irregularly addressed) or to Police Headquarters. I manage to read them all and have seen to it that they were adequately answered. They represent a large cross-section of the unhappy overweight masses, many actually pathetic.

Each letter, without exception, was from a diet failure, who had hopefully tried "all ways" not only to lose weight, but to keep it off. Many had tried semi-starvation methods. These also failed. Many had taken the various appetite suppressors, which had succeeded in only producing extreme nervousness and irritation.

They spent considerable sums of money on advertized "sure-fire, proven" methods, which only proved to be a sure-fire way to relieve them of much hard cash.

Each letter described essentially the same pattern. Most all of the writers had gone through the usual testing, and as expected, were told the same story. "See, your glands are normal. You just eat too much." No one believes them when they said they did not eat that much. This letter writer from Pennsylvania tells the story of that offhanded treatment.

"I have been reading in the paper about the cops losing all that fat. I weigh 230 pounds . . . P.S. I had an operation. My surgeon told me I was in good condition but go home and quit eating."

Every single letter contained a reference to the "little gray pills" (as the police and the newsmen called them). No matter how many inaccuracies about the function of the pills were published, every letter writer asked about them. One immensely overweight lady from Oklahoma said:

"Dr. I am volunteering to take off weight if I can get your help. If you send me the little gray pills I raise my right hand to God to take them like you tell me to."

The great majority asked if their own physician could obtain them or could prescribe them. This is a very heartening point, because, as I have already pointed out, if you need or wish to try the Supplement, your physician's cooperation is needed. Obesity is not a simple matter and should not be a "do-it-yourself" game in company with a group of amateurs.

One letter from an army colonel's wife, who was with her husband in South Korea, exemplified a certain pattern among many letter writers. She had ready the story of The Boston Police Diet and Weight Control Program in the Army's newspaper, *Stars and Stripes* and had written me immediately. Her letter was a recital of her efforts to lose weight at each new duty station. At some clinics the message was, "You are not a glandular case . . . you just eat too much," followed by the familiar advice about cutting down on calories. According to her letter, she "has been on more trial medications than any one she knows." My attention was riveted on one particular paragraph, which struck a very familiar note. This writer said that despite large doses of thyroid *hormone,* along with a 350 calorie daily intake, she not only did not lose weight, but she became extremely weak and irritable.

Herein lies the big mistake frequently, and perhaps inadvertently, made in many cases. Let me explain this to you. Using large doses of the metabolic hormone causes an acceleration in the functional machinery, much as stepping on the throttle of your automobile will increase the engine's r.p.m.'s. This leads to increased wear and tear on the moving parts. As the increased metabolism uses up more protein-derived tissues, more protein should be supplied to make up the wear and tear ratio. Now, it should be very obvious that with a 350 calorie diet . . . or even more than double that . . . not enough protein is being supplied to do much making up for the wearing out factor involving the combustion and utilizing mechanism. As a result, the apparatus is less and less efficient, which means that less and less of the fuel available is going to be ignited and burned. *If large doses of the metabolic hormone are used, increased amounts of protein must be supplied.* This was not done in the case of the colonel's wife and can often account for similar diet failures.

I earnestly hope that most of the letter writers are reading this book, and I also hope that they will have their own physicians prescribe the Supplement for them in the proper small doses along with a generous intake of protein. I believe that some very pleasant changes are going to take place among a lot of the former failures. Their cries for help have been heard.

Another frequently told story is the one that starts out: "I began to gain weight as soon as I stopped smoking." It's really absurd to put the blame there, but let's talk about it a little.

Smoking has NO action on body fat. It doesn't keep one from gaining, nor does discontinuing smoking account for the new accumulation of fat. Your "friendly" carbohydrate is still the villain. Listening to a lot of people you might get the idea that there are no fat ones among smokers, and they gain weight when they stop.

Let me make this point again. There are those individuals who will not become fat no matter what they eat or drink. On the other hand, there are those who can become fat if their carbohydrate intake exceeds their metabolic capacity. If these "can become fat" ones do not gain while smoking, it is simply because the cigarettes replaced their sweet taste. So instead of a doughnut or sweet roll, they light up another cigarette. But when, for any reason, they stop smoking, a substitute escape is needed to replace the "smoking fix." Let's assume that a person will drink more coffee or tea, etc. in an attempt to fill the cigarette void. With more coffee breaks there still is no source of fat accumulation . . . until sugar is added. Then there is the rationalization "Who drinks just coffee?" Ha, now it becomes "coffee and," which brings into the act such coffee companions as doughnuts, Danish pastry, sweet rolls, cookies, cake and in fact, the whole family of pastries . . . and perhaps even the sandwich with its inevitable two slices of bread.

So we have shot down the fattening powers or non-fattening powers of cigarettes. It is the old nemesis . . . the carbohydrate. Food still remains the most prevalent, but pleasant, addiction. It's just too bad that the wrong ones are addicted to the wrong foods. Please, stop blaming your weight gain on the fact that you stopped smoking. If you are putting on excess fat, blame the real reason, which is that you are now taking in many more carbohydrates than you formerly did, when perhaps the cigarettes took the place of some of the carbohydrates.

EXERCISE AND THE OVERWEIGHTS

The subject of exercise never fails to produce a lively hassle among the proponents and opponents . . . each sure of his own position. However, to avoid such a hassle, I am going to confine this chapter to the role of exercise in obesity. I may cross the lines a few times since the subject of exercise has many disputable points.

First, it should be accepted that exercise alone is NOT going to influence weight loss. The average amount of energy expended during even prolonged exercising will convert to an amount of heat that is totally insufficient to burn off any fat. Citing statistical figures, someone has worked out the formula that it would require at least sixty or more miles of steady walking to burn up one pound of body fat. This does not refer to the pounds of weight lost through heat evaporation (sweat) which are promptly restored with fluid intake. Even more vigorous exercise will do no more, since it is, at best, confined to a relatively short period of time.

No one ever lost weight through exercise alone without some dietary adjustment. Usually, if the food intake is restricted enough, the increased physical activity will require fuel to supply the energy needed. If little fuel is provided from the outside, then body fat will be the major source of energy as a fuel. Yet if the fuel (fat) is not ignited and utilized, the exercise becomes a tiring effort. Building muscle is the goal of many who must be reminded that in order to build muscle, one must supply the material from which it is built. This inevitably leads back to the necessity for protein. If a diet is so restricted that only very small amounts of protein are included, the need for protein may far exceed the amount supplied and result in "cannibalization" of the body's own protein tissue. This amounts to starvation, which is certainly not likely to contribute to good health and functional efficiency.

Any exercising overweight individual who does not supply any appreciable amount of carbohydrate but does supply protein will then burn the only fuel available . . . the excess body fat . . . providing the protein intake is completely utilized. If your igniting level is deficient enough, the body fat is not going to burn off, especially since the protein intake will have to be restricted sufficiently to fit within the deficient igniting and utilizing level. It's quite a merry-go-round when you really understand the machinations. The more exercise you want to do, the more protein is needed. But what good is an increased protein intake if it cannot be completely ignited and utilized?

The Supplement would be the needed extra spark to ensure better and quicker results in these cases. It might surprise you to find out how many exercisers on restricted diets tire so easily and cannot continue with their planned exercise programs. It all boils down to this simple fact: the more you use your muscles, the more you need protein (muscle material) to resupply that used during the inevitable wear and tear phenomenon.

Just picture this. Overweight persons with excess body fat waiting to be ignited and utilized arise in the morning . . . the entire day ahead of them. The energy requirement begins at the start of the day. Since they already have the source of the energy (fat) piled up on their bodies, no other fuel need be looked for. Only protein is required to keep the utilization apparatus functioning efficiently. Naturally, the igniting capacity must be also considered, but what is provided in that breakfast? Some grapefruit or orange juice, which at best provides a small amount of natural sugar along with the water and pulp. No protein is provided at all. The black coffee is merely coffee flavored water and no source of protein. Thus, the morning is actually lost. When noontime arrives (even then an adequate supply of protein would greatly help, even though the preceding hours were barren of energy production) all they are allowed to eat is a small scoop of tuna or a single small hamburger, scarcely adequate protein intake. The evening meal isn't much better. Another small portion of meat, chicken or fish is allowed, along with some green vegetables (no protein there). If that individual loses some weight, it is most likely due to some body tissue (protein) loss or starvation. Weight loss does not always mean fat loss. It can well be protein tissue breakdown loss. How long do you think anyone is going to stick to that type of diet?

Now, suppose the individual did some exercising. This will mean more wear and tear on protein tissue, which will NOT be compensated for. With or without exercise, breakfast should be treated as the first demand for protein of the day.

Exercise is only as good as the daily adherence to it. Tiring exercise is the wrong type of exercise. I'd rather use the term physical activity which more naturally seems to include walking, bending, turning the head, rocking, even opening and clenching the fist. The degree of activity you're used to is very important, as is your age. Obese middle aged people should not start a program of physical activity or vigorous exercise alien to their daily schedule. Let the younger ones do it . . . if they like. Everyone must learn the importance of daily adherence to a normal degree of activity. Obesity and premature aging (heart attacks in the relatively young) are NOT normal, and in my opinion, are not going to be actively influenced by diet or exercise alone. The key to premature aging or obesity lies in a hereditary metabolic disorder. This is why I have strongly advocated the daily use of the Supplement, trusting that the premature changes *have not passed the point of reversibility.*

"Moderation is the silken string running through the pearl chain of all virtues." If only those middle-aged, obese joggers and gymnasium enthusiasts had thought of the above line, it is quite likely that disaster would not have come to them. Usually sedentary men need not radically change their physical activity routine in the hope that new good health and better hearts are going to be theirs. Everyone has to do some walking during the day, so just add some more to it. This isn't in itself going to make you lose weight faster, but it will help to keep many muscles in better tone and to keep you away from food longer (the wrong foods around the house are too tempting . . . so go out more).

There is nothing special in bicycling that can't be found in regular walking habits. In fact, you are much less likely to give up walking than riding your bicycle. It always comes back to the same qualifications: do the kind of exercise you can do year after year with the least inconvenience . . . and the most regularity. Not exercise but dietary adjustment enables the excess body fat to become utilized. The running or vigorous exercise cannot and will not have any real effect upon an existing metabolic disorder. Most of my patients who are taking the Supplement don't bother with running, jogging, or any special exercises. They eat well, but correctly, and do not engage in any physical activities outside their usual daily established habits.

The daily workout has become a virtual fetish with the members of the body beautiful cult. Each day they faithfully perform the ritualistic weight liftings, push-ups, clockwise and counter-clockwise gyrations . . . usually resulting in a build up of the muscles involved. But why the build up? If they were in training for an athletic contest involving these exercises, then I could see and understand the reason. But to sit at a desk or to perform other routine occupational tasks, muscle build up is scarcely a necessity. Unfortunately, too many of these individuals who boast about being in good shape are also quite reluctant to admit how tiresome these demanding daily exertions have become. Still they force themselves to continue, knowing full well that the state of being in good shape depends upon continuing these same exertions day after day. Eventually, when the inevitable occurs and the daily ritual becomes irregular or even ceases, the good shape goes on a downhill slide. No matter what type of exercise program you embark upon, the guiding condition should always be . . . is it something that I can do safely and conveniently, day after day, without tiring myself? Vacationers seeking a change from their daily routines frequently are attracted to resorts because of the many activities offered. Some of these same individuals who came to relax . . . and what goes with it . . . soon find themselves hard put to keep up with the many physical activities planned by the director. Many eventually force themselves to compress everything offered into their two week period. No one wants to miss anything, and the hours of rest become shorter and shorter. When finally the vacationer returns home, he needs a rest period to recover from his vacation. This may sound a bit exaggerated, but I don't think it is. I'm not shooting down the resorts. Rather, I'm critical of the poor judgment used by too many of the wrong ones, trying to do things that they really aren't up to. Exercise should not be tiring. Professional athletes are, in my opinion, gross violators of this sensible advice. Because of the seasonal aspect of most sports, many start getting in shape only shortly before their season starts. This usually means vigorous, concentrated physical efforts in a relatively restricted time period. Some with a weight problem (oh yes, athletes can have weight problems) have to resort to a period of virtual starvation in order to "make weight" or to get rid of some accumulated excess body fat that was acquired between seasons. I have been consulted from time to time by various professional players, or their advisors, for help in overcoming their overweight situation before the season begins. I recall one case in particular, a well-known football player, who, as he informed me, had a weight problem as long as he could remember. Between seasons he would live the good life . . . eating and drinking the wrong things, then, when spring practice began he was put on reducing diets totaling no more than eight hundred to one thousand calories. He would omit breakfast (because practice started late in the morning and continued until late afternoon) as well as lunch. Then, at evening meal time, he felt entitled to make up for the earlier meals missed. This type of misguided nutritional schedule resulted in some interesting and near-disastrous patterns.

Firstly, he did not lose weight usually, despite the physical activity of his game. Secondly, he played a game which demanded much energy output, which he woefully lacked.

I spent considerable time explaining why and where he was so totally wrong. It was the same story I have outlined repeatedly in this book. How can one expect energy when the source of it is either not available or not utilized? He had the source available in his excess body fat at the beginning of each day. That fat or fuel was just waiting to be ignited and utilized. But if there was no breakfast, obviously there was no protein. It is no surprise that energy was lacking. Not only did I start him on a steak and eggs breakfast, but also to ensure his fuel utilization and igniting factors, I gave him the Supplement every day. The results were akin to a fictional story. He was awarded the "Best Comeback Player of the Year" title. I believe that if your livelihood involves a type of effort which demands certain standards, the dietary and allied schedules should be consistent all year round. I don't believe in annually getting into shape for your seasonal activity. Fighters are notorious for letting down training between fights (particularly those who fight infrequently) and then going on a rigorous and sometimes exhausting training schedule to "make weight" for the event. If you learn to eat correctly, there should be no need to let your guard down in eating and drinking habits. Steak, for example, is important for more than the training table.

All this should be of interest to the sedentary types, who, after approximately fifty weeks at their accustomed work, literally knock themselves out trying to become athletes at some resort.

SCALES AND CALORIES

Forget about scales and calories for the present. Right now it's much more important that you familiarize yourself with proteins and carbohydrates. Scales do not produce excess fat on your body

. . . nor do they help to get it off. Right now is the time to recognize the source of body fat and to make the adjustments which are recommended in this book.

No one ever became fat from proteins. Keep this fact in mind. The source of body fat is carbohydrates and all the scales in the world cannot alter this. If you are accumulating excess body fat, the message is quite clear.

A weight increase on the scale can be due to other factors besides fat accumulation such as increased muscle mass, increased bone structure . . . even putting weights in your pockets. Let the increase in clothes size be your weathervane and accept the fact that excess fat accumulation is responsible for the increased size. As the excess fat is lost by burning it off, your clothes size will change accordingly.

Weighing yourself constantly presents another problem. Since fat must melt before it can be excreted, you might get on the scale at the wrong time, before you had excreted all of the fat that was beginning to melt. You would be surprised and perhaps disappointed that you hadn't lost more.

Let me give you an example of the scale's inability to give you a true gauge of fat loss. Suppose you ate a one pound steak. After you had eaten the entire steak you would have gained one pound (the weight of the steak). You would have to get rid of an equal pound of something to bring your weight back to what it was before you ate the steak. Since the steak is mostly protein and doesn't burn up, but instead converts mostly to repair material for the tissues which are undergoing wear and tear, you would have to get rid of one pound of something else to keep the weight the same as before. This something else would be your excess body fat, which is the only fuel available for burning, as long as you do not supply any carbohydrate from the outside. Since carbohydrate is ordinarily a quick burning fuel, it would take precedence over the body fat fuel and thus detract from the amount of fat which could be burned. If you did not add any carbohydrate and the scale showed the loss of the one pound gain from eating steak, it would mean that you burned and excreted one pound of your body fat.

If this seems somewhat complicated, let me put it this way. Suppose you weighed 150 pounds. After eating the one pound steak theoretically you would weigh 151 pounds. If later the scale showed your weight was back to the 150 pounds, it would mean that one pound of burned body fat was excreted to offset the added one pound increase from the steak. If the scale read 149 pounds, it would mean that you had gotten rid of two pounds of fat, off-setting the pound of steak plus another pound lost. This means that you will have lost two pounds of fat, even though the scale shows only one. But your size will have changed according to the amount of fat being burned and then excreted through the urine.

This is why I always ask each patient before they get on the scale, "Are your clothes fitting any differently . . . or looser?" Suppose a patient says, "I must have lost weight. My clothes seem much looser." But the scale shows no weight loss. You can't take back what you said before getting on the scale about your clothes feeling looser. This only means that at this particular weighing, although some body fat had already softened, which accounted for the looser feeling, not enough had completely melted to be excreted through the urine to offset the weight of the food and water intake up to that point. Yet the same scale, a day or so later, can suddenly show several pounds weight loss. This is why I discourage daily weighings. They are not a true indication of your daily progress. Let your clothes size changes tell you; the scale has to catch up sooner or later.

And while you're ignoring the scale, don't torment yourself with calorie counting. Just be sure you aren't eating the useless carbohydrates. All foods have caloric value. If they didn't, they couldn't be food. The calorie only represents the potential of energy in a specific item and if this item is not completely utilized, the unused amount of energy is then measured in calories not realized. If it is carbohydrate that is not completely used up, the caloric value of the unused portion does not convert to fat. It is unused or incompletely used carbohydrate that will convert to fat. "Sticks and stones may break your bones, but calories will never fatten you."

Malnutrition and starvation are too often defined according to the total daily calorie intake. Distinct differences, however, do exist in these nutritional deficiencies. According to various nutritional tables, individuals require a specific number of calories in their daily intake, according to their ages, sex, and type of activity. A minimum number is listed as the lowest acceptable level. Anything below this would be considered insufficient and very likely be termed malnutrition. This classification can be highly inaccurate because there are very many obese individuals whose calorie intake is much greater than the recommended total, yet they are victims of malnutrition. The calorie intake may be much more than the average, but the bulk of the calories are found mainly in one group . . . the carbohydrates. There is a totally inadequate amount of protein, despite the high calorie intake, which can result in pronounced malnutrition. I'm sure that you can now see the vital difference between malnutrition and starvation. A totally restricted calorie intake in all food groups produces starvation.

So we are back again to the same formula. It's not how many calories you consume, but the groups from which the calories are counted. In starvation or semi-starvation the lean tissue (muscles) goes more quickly than the fat. We don't want this, and it can only be avoided by adequate protein intake. High starch diets are conducive to malnutrition. They should be replaced by diets high in protein. We have used the daily Supplement to ensure the complete utilization of sufficient protein. If you can utilize only a small amount of protein normally, then your physician should consider the daily addition of the Supplement in order to help you in utilizing an adequate amount of protein. While the problem of weight control or fat accumulation is usually a permanent one, calorie restricted or semi-starvation diets cannot be followed permanently.

SOME WEIGHT-LOSS EXAMPLES

Since most diet books have considerable space devoted to examples of "alleged" spectacular weight losses apparently to dazzle and impress you, I shall suppress my inherent modesty and just list a few progress reports from my case histories, both BPD program members and private patients. Though some lost at a quicker rate than others on the same program, two factors must be noted. Everyone lost weight, and everyone was taking the Supplement daily. You will read elsewhere in this book of the importance which I attach to this Supplement, not only because it may make the difference between losing and not losing, but, specifically, its role in retarding premature hardening of the arteries (premature aging). And I must note again: *no heart attacks* have occurred on this program.

Here are some weight-loss examples from the BPD membership list:

Patrolman F.G., age 33, always had a weight problem. Also, he had significant high blood pressure when first examined.

	Starting	
September 27, 1965	weight:	260 pounds
October 11, 1965	weight:	248 pounds
November 15, 1965	weight:	225½ pounds
March 12, 1966	weight:	212 pounds
July 5, 1966	weight:	203 pounds

From March to July his weight fluctuated. The transgressions (dietary) responsible for the interference in weight loss did not discourage me since he merely yielded to the inner yearnings of the average fat one. I did not have him shot; instead, I leaned on him a little harder. I don't expect eating or drinking habits to be changed overnight. Yes, eventually, I do expect the change to become second nature.

Patrolman F.G. continued to stay at the 200 pound level until November, 1966, when he finally broke that barrier and reached the 190 pound mark. At present, he fluctuates between 180 and 185 pounds. I do not encourage him to weigh himself often, but, instead, to get cracking if his uniform begins to feel tighter. This always allows for a few pounds either way without actual size change. His maintenance weight is in the 180's.

Captain R.C. started the diet on January 12, 1968. Starting weight: 245 pounds. He learned to eat steak or hamburger with eggs for breakfast and had to cut through former habit of cereals, doughnuts, and sugar. Weight May 8, 1968: 198½ pounds. Scale loss: 46½ pounds in 4 months.

Patrolman A.D. started the diet on January 13, 1969. Starting weight: 231 pounds. May 29, 1969: 185 pounds. Peak loss: 46 pounds.

Patrolman J.C. started the diet on March 18, 1969. Starting weight: 245 pounds. July 3, 1969: 200 pounds. Peak loss: 45 pounds.

Here are some spectacular weight losses among my private patients:

M.S., age 28, is a college professor. He was a most disillusioned and unhappy fugitive from several "easy weight-loss diet plans." He found it "quite illogical to literally starve while carrying a calorie bible to guide my daily starvation." His faith in various diet groups had been severely shaken. Reading one of the BPD press releases concerning the Program led him to my office as a private patient.

He first listened attentively to my two-hour orientation lecture. His comment, "I never knew these things about my problem before," I hear very frequently among my patients. Since he admitted to having been considerably overweight since early childhood, he was visibly shaken to learn about the important role played by heredity in obesity.

Perhaps a more detailed report of his progress will serve to encourage others who believe that their problem is actually hopeless, and that they must just "learn to live with it." If you are one who feels that way, just read on.

M.S. was first seen by me on July 24, 1969. His weight was 265 pounds. He was given a starting dose of the Supplement and urged to eat steak or hamburger for breakfast, with or without eggs. The amount of meat was not restricted as long as no carbohydrate was included in his daily intake. His progress chart follows:

	Starting	
July 24, 1969	weight:	265 pounds
July 31, 1969	weight:	256 pounds
August 29, 1969	weight:	228 pounds
September 26, 1969	weight:	212 pounds
October 24, 1969	weight:	200 pounds
November 21, 1969	weight:	189 pounds
January 16, 1970	weight:	175 pounds

This happy loser was ninety pounds lighter at the end of some six and one half months. By this time I began stressing the need for more self-reliance with less frequent office check-ups. The weekly visits are very essential during the early months, but should not be allowed to become a permanent crutch. I believe that once you are able to get with it, you should be gradually on your own for longer periods. By March this same patient weighed 165 pounds, and since then I see him every few months. At present, he maintains a weight level between 155 and 160 pounds. Although losing approximately 110 pounds in a year's time is impressive, I am truly more impressed by the fact that he has apparently learned to keep it off. Usually, stories about big losers stress the number of pounds lost in a certain period of time, but rarely do you see or read any follow-ups on these same individuals. It's the keeping it off that really counts. This is why so many diet plans fail. They are just not conducive to permanent weight loss.

Another remarkable example is *S.B., age 41,* who I first saw on July 22, 1969. His starting weight was more than the three hundred pound limit of my scale. He refused to be weighed on a high-register scale elsewhere, preferring to wait until my scale was able to register his weight. He returned on July 29, and again on August 5, at which time his clothes had a looser fit. Then, on August 18, he stepped on my office scale. He weighed exactly 286 pounds, but still would not disclose his starting weight, which he admitted he knew. His daily breakfast followed a straight pattern. It consisted of a good-sized steak with eggs, plus some unsweetened grapefruit juice and sometimes two large hamburgers with eggs, and black coffee, artificially sweetened. His lunch usually consisted of tuna or salmon with lemon, sometimes with a green salad, and either tea or coffee. He drank water and sugar-free drinks freely. His evening meal was usually steak, alternating with hamburgers, chicken, turkey, or fish, although he apparently didn't care to eat fish often. He included a green salad with a dressing made from safflower oil, vinegar, herbs, and artificial sweetener. I urged him to walk as much as possible, but to still rely upon our dietary protein and the all-important Supplement.

His progress chart follows:

	Starting		
July 22, 1969	weight:	over 300	pounds
August 18, 1969	weight:	286	pounds
September 16, 1969	weight:	268¼	pounds
October 21, 1969	weight:	256½	pounds
November 25, 1969	weight:	242½	pounds
December 23, 1969	weight:	232	pounds
January 27, 1970	weight:	222	pounds
May 12, 1970	weight:	199	pounds

Sincere attention to the problems of the obese can be both satisfying and frustrating. So many individuals are erratic and unpredictable. They can reach peaks of elation, vowing never to return to their former gross state. Yet, inexplicably, they simply disappear, discontinuing office visits. Some, when found, will contritely return to my benign supervision. Sadly, others react much as a confirmed alcoholic or other type of addict and succumb to the songs of the carbohydrate sirens. S.B. had informed me, after his weight dropped below the three hundred pound mark, that he had been weighed on a platform scale before his first visit to me and had weighed close to three hundred and thirty pounds. Thus, I can account for a weight loss of one hundred and ten pounds. This means that S.B. had lost some one hundred and thirty or more pounds during this first year, not by tortured starvation or calorie counting, but by eating very well and having the the indisputable aid of the Supplement. I can only hope that he has maintained his weight loss level even though he has not returned. S.B., wherever you are, give me a sign. I worry about you!

I'm quite certain that these spectacular examples impressed you most significantly . . . as I intended. Oh, they are authentic enough, but I had a motive for showing these quick losers. Remember, it isn't how fast you lose, but rather, how you lose and what you lose. Let's look a little closer.

Well-organized solid fat doesn't just melt away overnight. It takes steady, reasonable utilization of accumulated body fat, which must first be softened and then burned or melted. The melted fat has to be excreted along with the urinary output. When one sees losses of thirty, forty, or fifty pounds in a matter of a few weeks, it should be understood that these are mainly blubber or fluid losses, not old organized fat. Usually, where there is such fast losing, it is quite safe to say that the weight gain was fairly recent. People who have carried around a generous load of excess fat for years do not, as a rule, get rid of it overnight . . . which is as it should be.

Significantly, it must be remembered that these losers did not accomplish their missions by starvation or restricted calories. It is essential for you to know that during dieting that approaches true starvation, the lean tissue (protein) loss is greater than the fat loss. Since insufficient protein is supplied in such restricted diets, the body actually eats its own protein. One requirement remains constant on the Boston Police Diet and Weight Control Program: your protein intake must be adequate. If "adequate" requires the Supplement to ensure it . . . then so be it.

It's keeping it off that counts. Most of my patients do. I have the usual fluctuating on-and-offers. It comes down to their eventually and permanently deciding to get with it. No one starves.

CHAPTER IV

The Susceptible Overweight

THE WHO'S WHO AMONG THE FAT FRATERNITY

I have tried to classify the overweights for this special Who's Who not on a social or financial basis, but rather on the basis of distinctive habits and behavior. Find your own category. Laugh if you like; it's good for you. But don't go into a slow burn (at least, not against me). You'll find that anger and sensitivity are closely akin. They too often make you contentious and when that occurs . . . there goes your reasonable try at losing weight. I have seen too many thin-skinned overweights who become so unreasonably suspicious of any remark made in their presence that they immediately become very anti-social. Their defeatist attitude soon influences their food selectivity and, before you can say Jack Calorie, they defiantly gorge themselves with the very same things they knew were fattening. Who's hurting now?

1. The BEER DRINKER. (This doesn't apply to the beer drinkers who never gain, no matter how much they drink. They, lucky guys, don't need our concern.) The fat beer drinker usually is a many-faceted creation, crowned (in a manner of speaking) by the well-known "beer belly." This is truly an awesome structure. Many men with this much-protruding accouterment automatically learn to adopt the military stance of pregnant women. This is a shoulders-back lean to compensate for the drag forward. People have been heard to remark about what ramrod straight posture some of these persons have. They don't realize that if this miiltary attitude was not assumed, the poor chap could be dragged forward by the weight of his stomach into almost a stoop.

Neither should we overlook the natural extras that go along with beer imbibing . . . pretzels, peanuts and popcorn. So far, it's been bad enough, but if he is socializing, the genial host or hostess will further provide sustenance in the form of cold cuts, cheese, or potato chips. The processed meat and the cheese isn't all that bad, but who wants to eat it that way? No, some slices of bread become necessary as the vehicle to bring the food to his mouth. Strike one for the bread.

Since we are on the subject, we cannot neglect the hot dog or the hamburger. Don't forget that I am your staunch supporter of hamburger meat or even frankfurter (not as high in protein as the hamburger), but shun the vehicle . . . that bundle of carbohydrate called the roll or bun.

I'm not merely singling out beer over other drinks, but face it, if you are a beer drinker and have the potential of becoming fat, then beer is one of the most fattening drinks of all. If you qualify for these conditions, be warned, you don't just cut down on beer, *you cut it out completely.*

2. The SOCIAL DRINKER. This is the person who says, "But I only drink socially." You can become just as fat socially as you can anti-socially, if you drink enough . . . often enough.

3. The ONE MEAL A DAY AT NIGHT EATER. This is the indignant person who says, "There must be something wrong with my glands. I only eat once a day . . . when I come home at night." I gently inform him that unfortunately his one meal at night more than likely exceeds what he might have eaten in three meals during the day, along with the fact that the one meal probably goes on unceasingly for a good part of the early hours before bedtime. He doesn't like to be told that the same one meal total, if divided into three smaller portions, could be better utilized by his igniting and utilizing system and that he has overwhelmed it with the entire total at one time.

Actually, if this person were to eat that one meal at the beginning of the day, instead of at the closing, he might have a better chance to use it up because he would be more active in the daytime. But, more importantly, he needs the energy at the start of his day, not at the finish and as he already has a good supply of fuel (excess body fat) available just waiting to be ignited, the protein intake is indicated in the morning. So, if you were going to eat one meal daily, at least remember that the best time would be in the morning. But who wants to eat just once daily in the morning? Why not divide the necessary protein into two or three intervals and have a steady source of energy functioning? Breakfast is still the most important meal for the overweights. They need the protein then to start the fat burning. It's too bad that most people are conditioned to eat their main meal at six o'clock or after. You can still eat your evening meal, but start the machinery functioning in the morning. The noon protein intake doesn't have to be much, if enough was provided in the morning.

4. The COUNTER GULPER. Many never have time to eat breakfast at home, but always manage to find time to stand at a counter either in a drug store or some chain establishment gulping down in their proper order . . . first, the semi-faith ritual of the juice (perish the thought that one might drink the life-preserving nectar at noon or at night) followed by two and three doughnuts with coffee or Danish and coffee or just plain old rolls and coffee. What a breakfast! Very little protein, if any, but plenty of carbohydrate in the dough and sugar. Even if the individual didn't have a weight problem and could fully utilize the carbohydrate, it still would provide quick energy for a short burning time. So it isn't surprising that these gulpers are hungry by mid-morning. Now comes the coffee break, which mostly means coffee plus the accompanying companions, doughnuts or sweet rolls again.

I think the picture is beginning to unfold by now. So learn to start your day with P-R-O-T-E-I-N. Give special attention to steak, hamburgers (with or without eggs), bacon or ham and eggs. If you like fish, eat it in the morning also. You won't be considered a pervert if you do.

5. The AFFAIR CIRCUIT GORGER. This tour includes particularly the weddings . . . receptions or dinners or both if the dear bride has hooked a doctor (money well spent) or a well-heeled young executive.

Besides the weddings, there are the graduations, engagements, confirmations, bar mitzvahs, anniversaries, plus all the other walk-along-the-table, multi-choice eating feasts. Guess who is usually concentrating her attention where the rolls, cakes, cookies, knishes, potato salad, ice cream are! Worse yet, if they also are providing free drinks, guess who is concentrating his attention on the imported beer! No need to answer. I know, because I was once one of them . . . the overweights.

WHO'S FOOLING WHOM?

Since I am not exactly unknown around these parts, amusing incidents become rather expected interludes in my daily life. I am often recognized by enterprising overweights. The locale presents no challenge whether it be the food market, a social affair, a business conference, or just on the street. Invariably, the "on-the-spot advice seekers" will stop me for quickie answers. While the faces differ, the questions are usually the same. Real productive spots are food markets and social gatherings. The script follows a well-established pattern:

"Oh, you're that Dr. Berman, aren't you? Doctor, I want to lose weight in the worst way (they usually pick the worst way, too). What can I do"? While the unjolly, fat-insulated dear is anxiously pouring out her troubles to me, her hands are busily packing a dozen or two sugar-coated breakfast rolls, plus some diet ice cream into her already well-laden shopping cart. Then I might find myself gently but firmly being nudged over to the frozen foods section, where some inappropriately named TV dinners are being added to the goodies already stuffing her cart. The one-sided conversation continues at full tempo as our heroine appears totally oblivious to the make-up of the labor saving contents in the "specially prepared in our own kitchens" packages. What chance had I to meekly point out the fried chicken with its crisp, carbohydrate batter or the mashed potatoes or the sugar-sweetened applesauce? What was the use of my trying to point to the bonus of a well-crusted pastry tidbit? Ah, but all is not yet lost. I find myself confronting a formidable array of soft drinks, where, triumphantly, my well-padded, unhappy overweight holds up a bottle of diet drink and proudly says, "See what I drink? I watch the calories just like the girl on TV with her two calories per drink." Thus, the storefront consultation abruptly comes to a close as her eyes suddenly spy some articles on special sale. I step aside as she deftly steers the cart to the well-populated sale area. I can't help but overhear her saying to another non-slim shopper, "This is a real bargain. They are usually priced twenty-five to thirty-five cents more. I must get some." By this time I have become numbly indifferent to her bargain-priced *raisin pies.*

Did you say, "He's just making that up?" Well, of such stuff are the fat ones made. Stories or incidents concerning weight gain or obesity are not fictional. The so-called humor is tempered with a grim sort of tragic misbehavior. This deluded woman is like those women found at the meat and "deli" departments asking the man behind the counter to make sure the meat is very lean, while she has already bought potato salad, bean salad, crisp, well-battered egg rolls or knishes to bolster the flavored yoghurt she is adding to her diet. Such mundane things as the flavored sugary preserve at the bottom of the yoghurt container, which will have to be stirred and incorporated into the plain yoghurt, do not detract from her diet dish.

With many women, the economic factor influences their food selections. This is not an easy matter to cope with. Some years ago I would go regularly to various chain store food markets on the nights when housewives came in with their husband's pay checks. The ordinary working man came home with a modest check. Yet it had to have a certain "elastic" quality to allow it to feed a household of several active children and the parents and to cover the other necessities. I was most interested in seeing how the mother managed the food supply with such limited resources. Even then when food prices were considerably less than today, the dollar would still buy only so much. So the mathematical logic was that the cheapest priced foods would provide more to go around for the least money. One thing remains constant: the starches were the cheapest then and the starches are the cheapest foods today. It was no surprise to me when the shopping carts were loaded with such stretchable items as spaghetti, macaroni, noodles, potatoes, baked beans, rice, corn, bread, doughy items loosely called pastry, breakfast cereals, sugar, evaporated or condensed milk and usually the cheaper cuts of meat which meant bone and fat with a minimum of protein.

This will give you an idea of the economic side of the food picture. Let's now look at the functional or physiological side. Many of these mothers were just plain fat. Many of the children were also just plain fat. But there were mothers who were not fat or overweight just as there were children who also were not fat. Initially it depended on functional questions. Does this woman have the potential to become fat? Does she have a deficiency in her igniting capacity which would limit her complete utilization of any fuel? If she does and has grossly exceeded that limit in carbohydrate intake, the accumulation of excess body fat was inevitable. The factors of economy did not cause her to become fat. The cause was already present . . . heredity. But the economic issue, unfortunately, swayed her judgment toward the cheaper foods . . . the starches and sugars. In her case, these were the source of the body fat . . . not the cause.

You can find similar food choices in many school lunch programs. It might prove interesting for you to read some of the weekly menus printed in local newspapers. The number of calories provided in the meal are comparable to the total calories in the foods bought by the mother with the limited paycheck. However, despite potentially impressive numbers of calories such as 2,000 or 3,000, the calories are mainly represented in carbohydrates and a state of malnutrition could easily exist. Unfortunately, it doesn't appear likely that twenty-five cent school lunches are going to contain steak, or roast beef or roast chicken along with green vegetable salads instead of the well-potatoed hash, frankfurters, bologna, creamed chicken, spaghetti, macaroni, noodles, sugared applesauce and baked beans. Oh, I know they say there's protein in beans, but there is also at least twice as much carbohydrate.

I am not a crusader (at least not a misinformed one, I hope), but I can't help feeling that for so many overweights or potential overweights, the so-called good from the protein in certain products is more than a little canceled out by the existence of a sizable amount of carbohydrate in that same product.

It can be quite frustrating or laughable (take your choice) to see and hear commercial benedictions over the virtues of fluoride in various dental products followed by other commercial benedictions portraying the delights awaiting children upon eating the "new" candies, cookies, small pastries for toasting, and cereals with English-speaking animals. A common bond exists among them all . . . sugar.

Quickie Don'ts for the Overweights:

The Sub Sandwich
Also known as the poor boy, or hero. It's actually a loaf of bread with "stuff" in between.

French Fried Potatoes and
Malted Milk Chocolate Drink

Often eaten with hamburgers. The hamburgers are fine . . . without the rolls. You can well do without the potatoes and oh, the M.M.C. Drink!

The "Breakfast-In-A-Drink"
It may have 230 or 240 calories. "Equal to two eggs and bacon," so they say. Take the two eggs and bacon. They don't contain sweeteners (carbohydrate, that is).

The "Dieters" Plate
Consists of vegetables . . . lettuce, celery, carrots, plus other low or calorieless items. There is no appreciable protein.

The "Innocuous" Sandwich
and Glass of Milk
Eat a good protein meal instead.

THERE ARE NO SEASONS FOR DIETING

Let me begin by saying this: what is fattening in the summer is just as fattening in the winter. No one should be influenced by social occasions, either. If you have a weight problem, no celebration is going to make carbohydrates any less fattening for you. I cannot visualize any type of affair, be it banquet, dinner, luncheon or any business conference at which you are forced at gunpoint to eat dessert, bread, rolls, potatoes, ice cream, candy or drink any fattening drinks. Don't be misled by the mythical "drinking man's diet"; there just "ain't no such animal." While I am not a social butterfly, I do get around, accepting invitations to various affairs at which food and drink are in generous supply. I have always found items on the diverse menus which I could eat. The faithful standbys such as steak, roast, chops, chicken (not fried in batter), fish, salads . . . even *fresh* fruit cups are usually present. If lobster is on the menu, have it boiled or broiled . . . and dip it in butter if you like. Avoid the baked creatures with the usual sweetened dressing or stuffing.

New recipes are constantly being offered in magazines, newspapers and cookbooks. All seem to vie with each other trying to tickle the taste buds. Read as many as you like. No one ever became fat from reading. But before you try any of them, don't just reach for your handy calorie counter. You don't need it. Find out if sugar is involved in the dish. If the titillating tidbit requires sugar or has other carbohydrate ingredients in it . . . forget it. If you must, amuse yourself with some of the little "gems" found in my book. They aren't fattening.

All of this good advice simply adds up to this fact of life: If you have the potential for becoming fat you had beter learn to live well . . . but on the right foods . . . permanently.

Each springtime marks the advertising pitch invariably showing pictures of shapely lasses in appealing bathing or beach attire reminding you that you had better get with it, if you want to wear a suit like the one shown. The message is: if you want to wear a suit like this, hurry to join the such and such club or salon or group, and then in "ten easy lessons" (or perhaps five hard ones) you too can have this shape. Let's forget for the moment that the pictures are usually of professional models, who very likely never had a weight problem and probably never will. Let's concentrate, instead, on the steam baths, sauna, poundings, and massages, and mechanical gadgetry which do not and *cannot burn off fat.* Some, no doubt, do lose some weight with these ministrations providing they eat a diet of cucumber slices on lettuce leaves. How long do you think anyone can continue with the steam, poundings, massage and the lower-than-low calorie diets? If this applies to spring and summer . . . then what about winter and fall?

We always come back to the "gospel" that I preach. The proper dietary and weight control program is one that you can follow indefinitely . . . not on a seasonal schedule. Your phyical activity also should be geared to what you can conveniently do all year round. Your need for protein will always be with you. It cannot be sidetracked by cucumber slices on lettuce or any other low calorie menus.

You should not have to eat differently because it's summer or winter. You should eat less only if your energy requirement is less. As long as you have any excess fuel on you (excess body fat), you will still need sufficient protein to keep the machinery functioning efficiently. If your igniting factor is more than just a little low, the added assistance of the Supplement may make the big difference.

EXPLOITING AN OVERWEIGHT SOCIETY

The French philosopher, Voltaire, an astute gentleman, once said: "Quackery was born when the first knave met the first fool." How right he was. The attractions of quackery have never been more appealing. For many it is the lure of instant riches or instant fame or instant love, but the instant dieters are the most receptive. The instant inches off or instant spot losing or instant weight loss lead the pack in attracting the eager, gullible ones.

The experienced exploiters know the power of vanity appeal, and though names will never hurt you, they can hit your pride. Women don't relish being called fat, so to soften the blow, and with an eye to business, they are called stout or buxom or even . . . "over-matured." Of course, all this deceptive name calling still doesn't alter the fact that the unhappy dears still require larger sizes.

But beyond the garment makers and sellers stand the hordes of commercial friends with their newly discovered gadgetry and specially designed diets for quick weight loss, or spot reducing. The sums of money eagerly spent for the various belts, rubber garments, electric devices, steam baths, "health clubs" and "miracle diets" are staggering, and you may well wonder what happened to the minds of these generous contributors.

Fat is fat, muscles is muscle and bone is bone. Only fat is the most frequent cause of weight gain. Naturally, in the growing years, increasing bone and muscle substance will account for an increase in total body weight. After maturity one should not try to decrease bone and muscle volume. It can't be done normally. Disease can destroy bone and produce wasting muscle, but who wants to voluntarily destroy bone and muscle? Apparently some do, when spot reducing means trying to reduce muscle volume in various areas where the increase was due to muscle . . . and not to excess fat. Since muscle is protein-derived, some spot reducers have deliberately almost removed all protein from the daily diet so that the body must cannibalize its own protein tissues to supply the needed protein. Sounds rather stupid, doesn't it? This constitutes deliberate wasting of muscle tissue, usually in a vain effort to produce lessened tissue volume in selected areas.

Allow me to preach to you (just a short sermon) on the pitfalls of succumbing to the glittering lures of quick results. I'm pretty sure that most of you didn't accumulate your excess fat quickly. You still followed a natural pattern (wrong for you, of course) of converting the unburned carbohydrate into a reserve pile of fuel (fat). You should not expect this fuel pile to suddenly react to magic combustion methods and literally melt away overnight. Even starvation requires time. I am not suggesting that every follower of the BPD Program is going to dawdle away the excess fat. There is not a set schedule of how many pounds anyone must lose each week or month. It's something else to average up one's total losses over a given period of time, providing the time period is a reasonable one. I have seen many who were slow starters, then increased their losses regularly and steadily. Others may start with sizable losses, then gradually change to a slower but regular pattern. Quick losses at the very start are *usually due to fluid loss*. It's much like squeezing a sponge which has absorbed a lot of water. The first squeezes release most of the liquid . . . then succeeding squeezes yield less and less fluid. Of course, the sponge tissue itself won't become any smaller. I have questioned many patients who had formerly been on restricted fluid besides their restricted calorie intake. Diuretics had even been prescribed for them on a daily basis by mouth, with shots every week or oftener. These same persons were, no doubt, happy and thrilled for the first few losses, but after the squeezing period was over, their losses slowed down completely, and they resorted to semi-starvation. The entire regimen was very illogical and could be quite dangerous. These same persons soon became shoppers . . . looking elsewhere for a new or different way to lose quickly! You could justifiably call this procedure a lucrative quick turnover for the diet specialists, who always seem to have plenty of replacements for the disillusioned patient. Many of my new patients were fugitives from these quick-loss palaces. I try to set reasonable time periods for progress assessment. Let's say what has happened at three months, six months or after a year. How many pounds have been lost . . . plus what changes have occurred in the over-all size. You can average the total any way you like, by weeks or months, but when someone says, "I am wearing clothes that I had been unable to get into for some years," that's more important than how many pounds were lost. Naturally, if one goes from a size 22 or 24 to a size 14 or 16 (regardless of the time element), the scale weight is not going to be the same as at the beginning of the diet program. Don't be impressed with how much faster someone else loses. Even if you are careful, people are not all the same. Obviously, if your igniting or sparking capacity is more than a little deficient, you will have to restrict your protein intake and the progress may be slower. These are the conditions in which the Supplement makes a conspicuous difference.

There should be no restriction of liquids . . . as long as there is no sugar added to them. The melted fat eventually is filtered out through the kidneys and excreted along with the urine. People like numbers, but should not be dependent upon them. For example, patients have told me about reading somewhere that eight glasses of water must be drunk every day. How the figure eight was arrived at I don't know. I merely asked, "What would happen if you drank seven and one half glasses of water or even eight and one half?" Lesser amounts of fluid often would probably be easier to swallow than larger amounts less often. What does matter is that you drink sufficient fluid to help flush out the kidneys. It has nothing to do with melting the fat. The fat must be burned.

Fear is always an emotion for exploiters to play upon. Fear of the unknown has been exaggerated in people's minds, particularly when any seeds of doubt are planted concerning the safety of foods. Such soothing labels as "Health Food," "Nature Food" and "Organic Food," are, no doubt, very appealing to the many health worriers, who derive a sense of protection from these ill-defined labels. I doubt that I really know what these terms actually mean. It seems to me that all foods are health foods, since nothing could be called a food unless it had health benefit . . . even if it converts to fat. Dried figs or molasses from a health store are just as fattening as those from a conventional store. The only difference may be that you might pay more for the articles at the health food store.

Another timely exploitation is riding on the coattails of the latest "word of the year" . . . and the word is PROTEIN.

As you now know, everything must be converted into a usable state. Any food, be it protein, carbohydrate or fat, must be processed before it can be of any value. This processing involves varied activity of enzymes, digestives, hormones, etc., before it enables the food or fuel to be finally utilized. As an example: you don't just drop some protein down your throat into the stomach . . . and that's it. It requires several hours for the process of conversion to be completed. Then, and only then, can the blood absorb the usable protein and carry it to the areas of the body where it is needed as replacement material. Most of the body tissues are made from protein as the hair expert on TV confidently asserts. What could be more natural than squirting on the hair some concoction which contains protein since the hair is protein-made? Says *he* . . . not I. Here is a very convenient bypass of the usual route of conversion which would require the ingestion of protein with the subsequent absorption by the blood which then nourishes the hair follicles. Since the skin is also protein-derived, why not just rub a chunk of meat on the skin . . . bypassing the conventional route? You answer that.

I'm not trying to be a crusader. If you like being "had," it's your affair. But I do want you to have a reasonable understanding of the mechanics of nutrition before you make any decisions. Gadgets, health foods and instant anything will not affect how the food you eat is ignited and utilized.

CHAPTER V

Obesity and Your Health

OBESITY AND FUNCTIONAL SEX PROBLEMS

THIS is not a sexually oriented chapter about things you didn't know until now. The subject of obesity is big enough (forgive the pun) without adding sex counseling. Yet, I cannot completely ignore the physiological and psychological aspects of obesity. The endocrine glands can play a vital role in this area of metabolic disorder.

The term endocrine applies to certain organs or glands whose actual function is to secrete into the blood certain substances which play very important roles in metabolism. There is a sort of chain-hookup between these glands. What affects one can affect others . . . with most important end-results. Since this book repeatedly refers to metabolism, and the various disorders affecting it, I shall try to put the sex-obesity combination in its proper perspective.

A not uncommon situation exists among overweight or obese females in which they are apparently unable to conceive no matter how hard they try. Pregnancy just seems to elude them. I have seen considerable numbers of these disappointed and depressed wives, who were all the more bewildered since various tests had shown no apparent reason for their infertility. Yes, the husbands had been cleared also. It was called just one of those things . . . a conclusion which assuredly didn't help the already depressed subject. Yet something did happen among various females who had consulted me, or had been referred to me for their obesity problem only. Patients who had been given the metabolic Supplement as a part of my prescribed treatment not only lost weight as expected, but a significant number also became pregnant. I must hasten to add . . . not because of me . . . but because of the Supplement. Let me remind you again that simply losing weight by dieting alone does not affect an existing deficiency in the metabolic sparking substance. Apparently, since the thyroid substance along with pituitary and ovarian substance have a common relationship, a deficiency of the thyroid substance could contribute to functional infertility. There are ample numbers of females who did conceive after taking doses of thyroid substance. This must not be overlooked, since the tests (including metabolism tests) were all essentially normal.

Interesting statistical information cropped up when I did research on this project. Pregnancies do occur in women well past the usual menopause age bracket. Yet according to my digging, this rarely occurs to an obese woman past middle age. These same women were, in the main, never obese even during their younger years. Then, again, when a past-middle age male fathers an infant, rarely is he one of the fat ones. I still contend that habits do not account for longevity, despite the credit many old-timers attribute to such habits as chewing tobacco (since a boy), drinking strong booze or riding bicycles. The *hereditary pattern sets the stage*. As the thyroid decreases in size with age the secretions or output also decrease. If an old timer is still sexually active, you can be sure he has a more active hormonal output than is usual among senior citizens.

Let's move on to the psychological effects of obesity and sexual behavior. First, you would do well to dispel the ancient myth that fat people are the jolly ones. I have never quite understood why Santa Claus has always been portrayed as a jolly fellow with a big belly. Of course, I have never met the gentleman, but I should very much like to ask him if he enjoys having his faithful "steeds" struggling to pull not only a vehicle filled with toys, but also an obese, red-cheeked, white-whiskered old man sporting a belly of awesome proportions. I'd also like to ask him how he manages to squeeze that belly up and down chimneys of all sizes. Lastly, I'd like to ask him, "What's there for you to be so jolly about?"

Another case in point . . . the Merry Wives of Windsor (Shakespeare's creation). Who said they were all that merry? Singly or collectively . . . what did they have to really be merry about? Their obese lovers and husbands who appear to have derived great orgiastic satisfaction from gnawing on huge joints or drumsticks? By the way, I'm sure that they didn't accumulate their more-than-generous broadsides from the meat (protein). Bread and ale were much in flower then . . . along with knighthood.

Perhaps someone should compose a ballad entitled, "Where Are All the Fat Lovers of Yesteryear?" Or could you visualize a love story, particularly when displayed on the cinema or television screen, in which you would be treated to the spectacle of two lovers ponderously struggling to overcome the handicap of generous accumulations of adipose tissue (just plain fat) that serve to keep both truly at arms' length?

Believe me, I am not being derisive about the fat people. I'm merely trying to add more substance to the question, "What have they got to be jolly about?" I well remember my younger days when I wore a snug 42 waistline and attended various social happenings in the role of a buck on the range. Who do you suppose I got for my dancing partner or date? Not the slim adenoidal beauties, but, naturally, the "jolly" big ones who were warming the benches on the sidelines. The expectant but forlorn expressions were eventually replaced by the jolly expression of stomach satisfaction as the oral gratification of an ice cream sundae, dripping with thick chocolate syrup and topped with a generous handful of nuts, soon replaced any earlier deeper yearnings.

The tragedy here is in the fact that these same stout ones couldn't take their eyes off of the slim ones who were eating the same kind of sandwiches and sundaes with apparent impunity.

Many of my overweight female patients have unburdened themselves to me during my attempts to find out not why they became fat, but what prompted them to find their solace in the wrong foods. Most of these were married women, many with children. Let's examine some of the cases involving women who did have children.

Bear in mind the fact that we are dealing with those who are already fat. Very few of these were like that at the time of their weddings. We are not mainly concerned with this group, since the husband was quite aware of the size of the package he was getting.

But the husband or groom who was enthralled with the image of his trim or well-structured bride apparently saw only this image during their married years together. As the wife's weight began to accumulate, changes in the husband's attitude also began to accumulate. Remember, I'm not writing a novel or advice to the lovelorn book, but I am reporting the stories of certain patients whose domestic lives were affected by their weight problems.

Perhaps some husbands don't mind a fat wife, particularly when the husband is fat himself. They may just make a good team . . . or it may be the thing about "misery loves company." But the majority were faced with a dilemma. I would ask what came first . . . the increasing intake of carbohydrates, perhaps to demonstrate the wife's skill in cooking and baking (the wrong things), or increasing social activity with careless identification of the fattening foods and drinks? This can very easily lead to the well-known "despair cycle" in which the unhappy wife, becoming more and more aware that her mate's affections are slipping away, begins to find inner gratification in substituting food for sex. The chasm between the partners widens with increasingly depressing results. Then when some of these unhappy overweight, loveless wives and mothers finally seek aid, they are completely ripe for the well-publicized promises of quick, effortless weight loss and other similar "magic." Those patients who have been disillusioned graduates of the magic schools and have consulted me have a lot to undo.

To repeat my oft-used phrase, you cannot rub fat away. Those who may have lost weight while on a physical exertion type of program, also were on restricted calorie diets. Thus, weight loss of this type, necessitating also a restriction of protein, unfortunately does very little to enhance the physical attractiveness. While the scale may show lesser weight readings, the wan expression, the protein-starved skin hanging loosely, the lack of energy and go-power, combine to defeat the original purpose. A scrawny woman is a poor substitute for a fat one.

So far, I haven't even made mention of the various aids to dieting. Call them what you will . . . "appetite pills," "pep pills," "will-power pills," or "speed," the unalterable fact remains, *they are stimulants.* If something make you "high," then "low" must inevitably follow. It is so easy to develop a dependency upon these little helpers. A nervous, stimulated, scrawny female is worse than simply a scrawny one.

This type of dangerous crutch has no place in the Boston Police Diet and Weight Control Program. I want you to eat, but only the right foods. You will have to choose these for yourself. There are no pills with selective powers. The ONLY medication used in our Program is the Supplement . . . where it is indicated and where its supplemental effect permits one to eat more protein. No one gets high on this . . . unless you can get turned-on by steak, hamburgers, chicken, turkey, fish and eggs.

Lastly, early premature symptoms of menopause onset, that is, the sudden abrupt cessation of periods among many obese females with unpleasant side effects of the sympathetic nervous system, have been favorably influenced by the addition of the Supplement used in our program.

During my history-taking of new patients, I always ask them when they really started to gain waight and what their best normal weight was at early adulthood. The female patients could be separated into the following categories:

A. Those who began to gain steadily before the onset of their periods or were always chubby children.

B. Those who began to gain after the periods were established.

C. Those who had been normal in weight until after the first or subsequent pregnancies.

D. Those who did not begin to gain weight until they reached their forties or fifties. Many of them had never been pregnant.

We could go into other categories, but let's investigate those listed. I must remind you of some of my earlier statements that some persons would not and could not become fat because of their fixed hereditary potential. But let's zero in on those who had or have this potential to become fat. Some factor must activate or trigger this. Among the females exists a specific triad or trio of interconnected glands . . . the pituitary, thyroid, and ovaries.

What affects any one of these can affect the others. Starting with the female child who already has the hereditary potential for obesity, the first triggering of these glands is the onset of her periods. The potential thus becomes active, and if sufficient carbohydrate is ingested by this youngster (in excess of her capacity), the excess body fat begins to accumulate. Her friend, whom she envies, can eat the same amount of the same items with impunity simply because the potential is not in her familial pattern. Many parents and others can wait in vain for the overweight child to "grow out of it."

Let's go on to the next category. Here we may have the young woman who has the potential, but it has not yet been triggered. Menstruation failed to trigger the functional pattern of metabolic disorder. But after marriage, the first or subsequent pregnancies did and with the increased carbohydrate intake, the friendly fat begins to accumulate. As I've said, perhaps she wants to demonstrate her culinary capabilities. She also envies her friend who can bake, cook, and eat the same fattening foods, but who does not gain weight.

Lastly, there is the group who never became pregnant and who maintained a normal waight until their mechanism was activated with the onset of middle age. These women speak of their "middle age spread" with an anguished smile. The ovaries are now involved . . . downhill . . . as the active function begins to slow down and die out. Thus the menopause is not the same for all. Women with the metabolic disorder remain the same through and after the menopause.

In instances of more than casual gaining, I have used the Supplement with very significant and beneficial results. I would call ths delaying premature aging. The sense of new vigor and even sexual rejuvenation, which many patients have reported to me, cannot be attributed to merely dieting. Specifically, the Supplement makes the difference.

RETARDING OR EVEN AVOIDING PREMATURE HEART ATTACKS

The number of premature heart attacks is increasing annually, but conventional measures have apparently failed to stem the tide. Diet changes, vigorous exercise, not smoking, have not improved the situation. Yet in the face of all this depressing information, I feel deservedly proud that during the six years thus far of the BPD Diet and Weight Control Program, not a single heart attack has occurred among any of the participants. And the majority of participants are middle aged . . . and obese (or were obese). Both of these make for a dangerous medical combination. I do not credit the diet itself as being responsible for these remarkable results. Something *more specific* is *involved* and will be explained in more detail.

Every human being ages with or without use. All functioning parts must sooner or later begin to show signs of wear and tear. This is to be expected and is accepted as normal, when occurring in late maturity. Hardening of the arteries is no surprise when seen in the later years of life. But when it occurs earlier or prematurely . . . even in youth . . . this cannot be explained away by blaming it on saturated fats or cholesterol in the diet.

A series of autopsies performed on young soldiers killed in Korea and South Vietnam revealed *advanced arteriosclerosis* in many of these young men. In particular, the coronary arteries already showed advanced changes which would ordinarily have indicated advanced age. These changes, no doubt, would have significantly affected the lives of these young men had they not had their lives snuffed out prematurely. Had these prematurely aging young people lived, they would very likely have been subject to coronary heart attacks, stroke or other complications of hardening of the arteries. They may well have had the attacks in their late thirties, or in their forties or fifties.

Surely, one cannot attribute this clearly demonstrated evidence of premature aging to a lot of fat in the diet. If anything, persons in that age category would more likely be candy and sweets eaters, not to mention smokers and drinkers. It would have been interesting to have known about their family history. I'm sure that many would have disclosed a history of others in that family, even a generation or so ago, who had suffered heart attacks at a premature age.

Despite all the well-intentioned advice about cutting out the saturated fats, giving up smoking, reducing weight, running and other forms of physical activity, *the death rate from coronary heart attacks continues to increase year after year.* Obviously, something more specific is required. I believe the answer is found in being able to *retard premature aging by supplying the vital hormonal component which is lacking in so many.*

I have used the Supplement for the past twenty-five years, not only for my patients, but for myself as well. This measure actually supplements a metabolic hormonal deficiency which can exist naturally in advanced age or unnaturally in hereditary premature aging.

I believe that eliminating the useless refined sugars, with their empty calories, is an important step to reduce the accumulation of excess body fat and to decrease its contribution to hardening of the arteries.

If you have a familial history of early heart attacks or strokes or diabetes, even without being overweight, I believe the Supplement can definitely reduce the chances for these manifestations of premature aging or metabolic disorder, as is involved in diabetes. The average diabetic has insulin, since the source of it, the pancreas gland, is functioning as is the thyroid. But the amount of insulin that is available is not produced in sufficient amounts by the pancreas. Thus supplemental insulin has to be used. The thyroid exercises a controlling action over the pancreas, and the same type of anti-body immunity observed in obese individuals has been identified in diabetics. There are more diabetics among overweights than non-overweights. There are more premature heart attacks among overweights than among the non-overweights (those who are normally non-overweight).

Some time ago I compiled a list from the death notices in the newspapers. The list was made up of men in their 30's, 40's and 50's, who had died suddenly of heart attacks. A significant fact was that many of these men had fathers who had also died of premature heart attacks. This is more than sheer coincidence and points strongly to hereditary metabolic disorders. It should be obvious that in the face of such inherited functional premature aging patterns, jogging, dieting, bicycling, and other exercises are not going to functionally affect a hereditary metabolic disorder.

The thyroid has great importance as the source of the "sparking substance." Even in the normal circumstances accompanying the normal aging process the gland atrophies or becomes smaller. A normal lessening of its output is expected and accepted.

Some interesting investigative work concerning heparin was done by some German scientists just a few years ago. Their work was related to the natural availability of heparin in the blood. Heparin is an anti-coagulant which prevents clotting or coagulation in the vessels. Without this substance, clotting would occur in the blood vessels as it does when the vessel is cut and exposed to the outside. Heparin has been and is still being given to patients who have an abnormal clotting factor as in coronary thrombosis and cerebral thrombosis. Without it there could conceivably be an abnormal clotting action with plugging up of the smaller arteries and veins. Particularly in coronary thrombosis, it has been an accepted practice to give the patient doses of heparin to reduce the clotting factor, thus encouraging a freer blood flow through the narrowed vessels. Often the cure has been worse than the disease since abnormal internal hemorrhaging has resulted from the excessive anti-coagulant action.

Heparin is made in the liver and is subsequently released into the blood as needed. The controlling mechanism is the thyroid. The investigators compared the heparin content in the blood of a group of older individuals. They found that the older group had less than half the heparin found in the younger group members. The significance of this should not be overlooked. It is obvious that the heparin *decreases* with age. Older individuals are thus more prone to clotting changes occurring in thrombosis . . . even naturally. My own impression has been that when abnormal thrombosis occurs in so many heart attacks affecting the younger adults, instead of giving heparin as a supplement, which still does not affect the control center, I would prefer the logic of giving small doses of thyroid as a supplement to the controlling mechanism. I believe this will help to continue the heparin output from the liver.

As I have already pointed out, diet alone, even with exercise and the other conventional recommendations, will not and cannot prevent the process of premature aging.

For example, many coronary heart attacks have occurred among the obese. Assuming the patient survived the initial attack and, because of his overweight, was put on a strict reducing diet. No matter how much weight might be lost, this did not prevent recurrence of coronary attacks in many. Still nothing had been done about the cause of premature aging.

Since all of the participants in the Boston Police Diet and Weight Control Program were obese and were (and still are) taking the Supplement, our no-heart-attack record points to the value of the Supplement combined with the proper dietary measures.

Recently, some papers were published on work done in veterans' hospitals with thyroid supplement in helping to prevent and reduce the incidence of premature hardening of the arteries in young and middle aged veterans. Their reports were encouraging.

Even now I have been reading new articles in medical publications, in which the authors are urging the use of thyroid supplement in treating diabetics. A fairly large study group of diabetics were found to have significant changes in the blood-sugar levels (which dropped to within acceptable limits) after taking thyroid supplement for a reasonable period of time. Glycosuria, or sugar in the urine, also disappeared . . . without the use of insulin.

I am pleased to read these new reports, which confirm my twenty-five years of using the Supplement.

Obesity should not be accepted or regarded as a separate entity by itself. Particularly in more than moderate obesity, the strong likelihood of a hidden metabolic disorder should not be ignored or overlooked just because of a normal metabolism test. The thyroid itself is an extremely vital center, yet, on the basis of tests which showed normal functioning, serious disorders separate from the gland itself are too often ignored. It is a good thing to remember that the trouble can be farther down the line from the gland itself.

My results over the past twenty-five years, now bolstered by some recent published reports, have convinced me that abnormal blood cholesterol levels (Hypercholesterolemia) and abnormal blood fats (Hyperlipedemia) can and have been reduced to within normal levels by the use of the Supplement.

Even in the absence of abnormal levels concerning these conditions, I would still continue to use the Supplement in all true obesity cases, not only to increase the utilizing and igniting factors, but as a prophylactic measure against the ever-likely complications mentioned. The dosage does not approach therapeutic or treatment strengths which might be indicated in true Hypothyroidism.

So I repeat. Diet plans, and gadgetry, cannot and will not have any effect upon an existing metabolic disorder of hereditary background. They have still not reduced the ever-increasing numbers of premature heart attacks . . . despite the number of pounds lost. This same conclusion applies to the supporters of exercise, no smoking, etc., as measures to avoid heart attacks. Despite their beliefs, non-smokers have heart attacks as do athletes, particularly in the middle age bracket. Reducers still have heart attacks . . .

despite the removal of all fats from their diet. I am not trying to put down exercise or not smoking . . . I'm just advising you NOT to count on these measures.

In an issue of "Consultant," the heart specialist Dr. Paul D. White has written: "Unfortunately, however, the search for conditions that may contribute to coronary heart disease has focused almost entirely on environmental factors. *It's my contention that heredity should share that limelight.*"

I have always maintained that a pre-existing hereditary familial pattern is NOT going to be materially influenced by social or physical habits. I cannot accept the concept that certain types have a predisposition for ulcers, because of tensions, business challenges, eating or drinking habits. The definition of an ulcer is an open sore or an eating-away process involving skin or mucous tissue. For example, hydrochloric acid is among the substances normally found in the stomach. Some regulating mechanism must be responsible for keeping the concentration of hydrochloric acid from becoming erosive. While aggravations, tensions, excess smoking, or indiscreet eating may be associated with an ulcer, it is very unlikely that these habits are going to affect the physiological regulating center. The symptoms of an ulcer can be aggravated by the above factors, but the predisposition for an ulcer was there before. Since the acidic concentration of the hydrochloric acid is increased in ulcer patients, it would appear to me that some disorder of the regulating system is involved. Again I must stress the hereditary factor.

The subject of heredity is a deeply complex one, which can involve tracing back through several generations. Longevity is a hereditary trait in many family lines. Mature aging goes hand in hand with slow wear and tear. Thrombosis and arteriosclerosis are certainly not unexpected in those individuals who are in their eighties and nineties.

Various risk factor tables have been compiled by diverse medical groups and research centers. Much stress has been put on habits such as smoking, lack of exercise, high cholesterol, faulty diets containing saturated fats, and obesity. Bringing up the rear is mention of heredity. I would take issue with these factors in their order. Heredity should be in the number one spot. Next should be obesity. The others are merely incidental. High cholesterol should not be listed or considered as a separate factor, since it is a mistake to blame the condition on faulty eating of saturated fats. The cause of the abnormal cholesterol levels is what counts, not cholesterol-containing foods. The body builds up the cholesterol; thus even in individuals whose diets don't contain fat, high cholesterol levels have been found quite frequently. Again, I would go back to the source of the problem . . . functional disorders in the regulating hormonal system. A recently promoted new anti-cholesterol medication contains a thyroid product called sodium dextrothyroxine. (It would appear that the thyroid is being discovered at last.)

THE OVERWEIGHT TEEN-AGER

I cannot accept the validity of certain special reducing diets . . . whether for teen-agers or any group of "agers." If an individual has the potential for accumulating fat, then what is fattening for adults can be just as fattening for teen-agers. It all depends upon exceeding that particular igniting and utilizing limit. Teenagers should NOT be exploited any more than any other group merely because of the sales appeal. Only in recent times has there been a growing voice of protest concerning the poor eating and nutritional habits of our population in general. While I do agree that the *sugar intake is totally excessive,* I cannot agree with any contention that the fat intake is also high. One thing is quite certain. Protein has been relegated to the back seat much too long in favor of the "easier-to-appeal-to" exotic tastes of sweets. The birthrate of new candy and pastry confections is very high and constant. No commercial appeals describing the "delights" of fish, steak, hamburger meat, and chicken are directed at the younger segment of the TV or radio audience. If there are, they must have slipped by me. The virtues of fluorides in dental preparations may continue to be dramatically presented by the proud TV fathers in the presence of coaches, golfers, fishermen, and otherwise occupied adults, who show not the slightest annoyance or resentment at being interrupted by an enthusiastic youngster's cries of victory over cavities. Of course, all within hearing distance immediately dropped whatever they were doing and, in unison asked, "How did you do it?" The superiority of fluoride was lauded and as an afterthought a small voice hurriedly said something like "limit treats." Unfortunately it didn't say, "Limit candies, pastries, ice cream, and sweet drinks." Apparently it is not necessary to go into any detailed explanations of what constitutes "treats." Rewards for good deeds are never openly confused with such mundane items as hamburgers (without rolls), steak, fish or fowl, but are invariably associated with some special type of pastry roll, which fairly drips with sweet gooey centers or some tantalizing candy product (regardless of whether it does or does not rub off in your hand).

Dear teen-ager . . . you may be thirteen or nineteen to qualify for this somewhat outdated label. I believe it was back during the days of "Harold Teen" and "bobby-soxers" that this title held forth. Today you are probably identified as "the young people," "the kids," "young adults," or "the youngsters." However, one fact remains constant, there have always been plenty of fat or overweight teen-agers. What was fattening yesteryear is just as fattening today. If you are one of those with a potential for becoming fat, the source of the fat remains the same . . . *the carbohydrates.* You don't need special books or reducing camps to do the job which only you can do. I won't bore you with such pseudo-impressive terms as motivation, conditioning, and self-analysis. If you really want to lose weight then remember that the excess fat didn't come from playing drop the handkerchief or post office. If you *give up the common sweets,* at least you should *stop gaining.* Then, emphasize the role of protein and eat hamburgers, steak, chicken, roast, eggs, and fish (if you like it). Give yourself a reasonable time to show some results. Don't make a race out of it. You have plenty of time to lose and to learn how to keep it off.

If you are certain that you aren't making any progress through reasonably changing your food intake, then you may need some help from the Supplement. Your physician should decide this since true obesity is NOT a "do-it-yourself" game. It should be accepted as a medical problem which can and frequently does involve a hereditary metabolic disorder. Don't jump prematurely to the conclusion reached by too many individuals that when the word metabolism is mentioned, the thyroid itself is always involved. If you have read the book thus far, you will surely have seen that the trouble may go beyond the gland itself. Thus it will be most important that you find a sympathetic and able physician to guide your efforts.

Let's go over a list of the frequently abused foods and drinks which you often eat and which are fattening.

THE NO-NO'S

All sugar sweetened soft drinks. Look for sugar-free. Candies. All varieties. There are no real diet ones. Pies. Cakes, Cookies. Doughnuts. In fact, *all* pastry items. Ice cream. Frappes. Sodas. Sundaes. Malted drinks. Batter-fried foods. Get it without the batter.

Spaghetti. Macaroni. Noodles. Rice. Bread. Crackers. Rolls. Sandwiches. Forget the two slices of bread. Pizza. All breakfast cereals. Especially the frosted ones. Too much milk. Flour-thickened gravies and soups. French-fried potatoes. In fact, all potatoes. Baked beans. Jellies. Jams. Preserves.

You'll survive without the ritual of a peanut butter and jelly sandwich.

I can appreciate the desperate attitudes of teen-agers toward being fat and being the targets of unsympathetic and unreasonable friends. I can look back some fifty years when I was in high school and because of an over-generous coat of excess body fat had to undergo the daily salutations of "Tubby," "Chubby," "Fatso," and the like from my classmates. I still remember the chocolate dripping down their faces from their candy bars and their malt and coke guzzling and feeling a sort of hate toward them because I just could not understand why they didn't gain weight eating and drinking the same things that I did. Even the common and frequent incidence of acne among so many of us was misunderstood and attributed to some mystical sin. As I recall, the fat teen society, of which I was a prominent member, had a greater tendency toward postular acne than did the non-members. Acne was misunderstood, but a greater misunderstanding existed about the role of sugar as a proliferant media for the staphylococcus organisms which flourished in the pus-producing by-products of acne. Today, acne is accepted as a phenomenon of adolescence, and along with other advice given, teen-agers are urged NOT to continue eating sweets *because* of the sugar. Since acne can be associated with metabolic changes at puberty or adolescence, even though it continues for an extended period of time, I have, with pleasure, noted favorable changes occurring among many of my overweight, adolescent patients who took the Supplement as part of their daily routine.

I never discourage physical activity for the overweight teens, but I also emphasize that activity alone is not going to affect the overweight situation without a change in food intake. So the dietary program is vital to all overweights . . . teens and adults alike. Eat more protein. If you drink milk, *don't drink so much.* There has been a tendency to overdo the milk thing. Whether or not it is whole or non-fat milk, the lactose (milk sugar) is still present. This can be fattening if enough is ingested. I would discourage the heavily advertised energy breakfast cereals. I'd still settle for eggs and bacon instead of the calorie counted bowl of fortified stuff. They forget to mention the 75 to 80 plus percent of carbohydrate content. Learn to read the labels on boxes or packages. Know what the contents really are. Don't just listen to the enthusiastic pitch. So, in conclusion, I would suggest that teen-agers become better acquainted with fresh citrus fruits, green vegetables, and above all with meat, poultry, and fish. No one ever became fat from these.

THE SUPPLEMENT: TO USE OR NOT TO USE

The goal of most overweights is to lose weight . . . the quicker the better. How it's done, unfortunately, does not concern the frantic fat one . . . just quick loss. So is it any wonder that so many of these unhappy, unthinking overweights eagerly respond to the lures of the "how to lose weight fast and painlessly" methods or groups? The turnover among these must be tremendous, judging by the rate at which new ones appear.

Let's look at this weight problem from my point of view. I'm sure that since you are reading this book you must have more than just a passing interest in the problem of obesity. Having once been overweight, I honestly believe that I can understand your feelings more sympathetically than the promiser of quick results.

If you think merely losing weight solves the problem, you are very mistaken. If the problem was simply that of overeating, as you no doubt have been repeatedly told, then truly it would be only a simple problem. Of course, this simplified solution leaves much to be accounted for. It fails to take into account such annoying questions as:

How much is overeating?

Is there a specific kind of food that I am eating too much of?

Does it mean that all foods are fattening if one eats too much?

Why doesn't my friend (or others) become fat eating the same amount of the same foods that I do (even more than I do)?

Why don't I lose even when I almost starve myself?

Why do I usually gain back the lost weight when I stop starving myself?

Do I have some kind of glandular condition even though my metabolism tests have been normal?

These are only a sampling of the factors which should be considered and explored when dealing with the overall problem of obesity. It just isn't a matter of losing weight by any means to produce that result. People are different. What is too much for one is not too much for another. If this functional difference is only minor, then as I have already explained, a sensible readjustment of your food intake is usually all that is required to stop gaining and to begin using up the excess body fat. The one constant condition is that carbohydrate intake be drastically reduced, particularly useless sugars, although the starches shouldn't be overlooked.

If, however, this measure does not produce results, and if adequate weight loss does not occur except through semi-starvation . . . then, it is wrong to continue along those lines. This plainly points to more than just a minor igniting capacity deficiency and is, in my opinion, a compelling justification for the use of the Supplement. The vital importance of sufficient protein intake has been repeatedly stressed, yet protein intake must be completely utilized also. A free intake will depend upon the volume and efficiency of the sparking and utilizing factor. For those with limited spark, the Supplement makes the difference between active losing and slow starvation.

I would say this to your physician. If your patient has been unable to lose weight except by an unreasonable restriction of all food and even this in some cases was ineffective, then consider prescribing the Supplement in supplemental doses only. If there is also a history of diabetes, premature heart attacks, hypertension, hyperlipedemia or high cholesterol in the family, I most certainly would prescribe the Supplement for any such patients of mine. The decision would be yours. All former diet failures are entitled to the strong probability of successful results.

I have used various thyroid products in former years such as triiodothyronine, and thyroxin, but for the past few years I have used only plain, uncoated tablets of thyroid extract. The strength and dosage depends upon the age and size of the patient. Usually for just moderately overweight patients I have started with one fourth ($\frac{1}{4}$) grain tablets three times daily or two $\frac{1}{4}$ grain tablets in the morning, one at noon, and one at 5 P.M. With the more stubborn cases, I use one half ($\frac{1}{2}$) grain tablets, three times daily or at most two half ($\frac{1}{2}$) grain tablets in the morning, then one half ($\frac{1}{2}$) grain tablet at noon and one half ($\frac{1}{2}$) grain tablet at 5:00 P.M. I have NOT had to use more than two grains total for a daily dose in any case.

Sufficient protein must be provided to equal the increased wear and tear resulting in the muscle tissue. As long as no carbohydrate is supplied, the excess body fat remains the only fuel available to burn.

I have had NO stimulative effects. Blood pressures, if high, have been lowered most favorably. The side effects frequently seen with the use of the appetite-suppressors or euphorics are entirely absent since they are never used . . . nor are they warranted. There has been a most gratifying reduction in any high cholesterol levels. Some of the new cholesterol medications contain sodium dextrothyroxine. It would seem that thyroid, as a supplement, is just being discovered. I have been prescribing and taking it myself for the past twenty-five years.

FOR THE PHYSICIAN: A SUMMARIZED DAILY SCHEDULE

If you wish to follow this operational guide for your patients, especially the intractable ones, the results should be quite favorable.

For the average overweight who is at least twenty-five or more pounds above the optimum weight, we start with the following dosage of plain uncoated thyroid tablets:

MORNING: One half (½) grain before breakfast. An adequate amount of protein must be provided. Steak and eggs, hamburgers and eggs, bacon and eggs, ham and eggs. (Eggs are optional although cholesterol levels have been normal while taking the Supplement).

NOON: One half (½) grain tablet. Protein again. Can have tuna, salmon, sardines (drain oil), cold roast, green salad.

5 P.M.   One half (½) grain tablet. Evening meal can include meat, fish, poultry, green salad. A cooked green vegetable is acceptable. Can have a half grapefruit once or twice daily or unsweetened juice.

If the patient is excessively overweight, we use two half-grain (½) tablets in the morning, then a one half (½) grain at noon. Finally, a one half (½) grain tablet at 5 P.M.

Patients are urged to drink plenty of fluids (coffee or tea without sugar), sugar-free soft drinks. No milk as a drink because of lactose milk sugar. Can put some in coffee if desired.

If the patient is excreting insufficiently, we use a diuretic twice weekly. My choice has been Renese (2mg. tablets). One half (½) tablet twice a week in the morning with the Supplement.

You use any diuretic you wish. I recommend small doses . . . infrequently.

A CONVENIENT SUMMARY

I would recommend that you read and re-read this summary from time to time. No matter how much you might assure yourself that at last you completely understand your weight problem and know how to manage it, you will be quite surprised to find out, at each re-reading, how much your understanding is increased. Small but important things which you missed during earlier readings have a way of cropping up.

Start having daily discussions with yourself concerning what you should and should not do.

The following principles should guide you on a day to day basis until they become permanent. You'll learn, if you haven't already, to bid farewell to calorie-counting bookkeeping and to trust your new knowledge about what is and what isn't fattening.

You'll know how much more important protein is than carbohydrates.

You'll know that all individuals are not the same. That their igniting and utilizing systems have varying degrees of total function. You'll also know how one individual can normally ignite and utilize more fuel than another, desipte their apparent similarity.

You'll know that there are countless numbers of fellow human beings who were literally "born to be fat," and most likely become that if given free rein in their eating habits.

You'll know that very few of these hereditary chosen have an actual abnormal glandular condition. Metabolic tests have proved this. The crutch of rationalizing by blaming all on a sluggish thyroid must be thrown away. You'll no longer need that phony psychological support. And better still, you'll know at last that too much for you does not imply huge amounts of food.

You'll know how well you can actually eat even with proper food choices. Once you have opened your eyes to the empty food value of so many fattening items that you once enjoyed and recognize them for what they really are . . . your sweet enemy . . . you will be on your way.

I believe that after reading this far, you can now well appreciate the importance of having your physician's cooperation in managing your medical problem, which is what obesity usually is, and forget the amateurs playing doctor.

1. Your major energy need begins with the start of your day.
2. The source of your energy is fuel. You don't have to supply it as it is already there. It is just waiting to be ignited and utilized.
3. Your excess body fat is the fuel you wish to burn, so don't add the other fuel (carbohydrate).
4. The apparatus involved in the igniting and utilizing process is all protein-derived. Increased operational activity of the apparatus will inevitably result in increased wear and tear of the working parts. In order to prevent wear and tear, exceeding the rate of re-supplying the material for the parts, enough protein must be provided to offset any loss of efficiency.
5. All of the protein must be utilized, thus if the igniting and utilizing capacity is inadequate, either less protein must be provided to keep within the limited capacity of igniting and utilizing or the reduced spark should be reinforced by supplemental amounts of the same substance. This allows more protein for more complete utilization with increased efficiency of the entire apparatus.

If you are taking the Supplement, take the first dose when you go in to wash. This way you have poured some fuel on your morning fire, quickly increasing the igniting power. The added igniting power will increase the operating rate of the machinery as it also increases the wear and tear on the parts. This is why enough protein should be supplied at this time . . . in order to keep up with the amount of wear and tear on the machinery. The efficiency of the igniting and utilizing factor will be kept at a high level as enough protein is supplied. As long as your excess body fat is the only fuel available, only it can be burned. Should you add some needless carbohydrate to your intake, then, quite obviously, the fat is no longer the only fuel available to burn and must share its exclusiveness with the carbohydrate. To keep you on the right track, let me repeat that I am not referring to the small amounts of natural carbohydrate in fresh fruit or unsweetened fruit juice (although even this amount should also be kept in check). I am plainly referring to the useless commercial or refined sugars in sweet rolls, doughnuts, cereals, bread, pancakes with syrup, waffles, jelly, marmalade, etc. These, even if taken in small quantities, can detract from the burning fat enough to slow down the melting process. We want your excess body fat to be the *only* fuel available for burning.

Now to get back to what you should eat: protein such as a generous portion of steak or hamburgers . . . with or without eggs, bacon and eggs, ham and eggs, fish (any kind, if you like it) or any cold leftover meat or chicken. Cottage cheese alone will not supply enough protein. Neither yoghurt alone. Watch out for the sweetened syrupy flavors. If enough protein is included in your breakfast, you don't have to eat more at noon, although you can if you wish to eat at lunch. If you eat lunch, divide the breakfast portion into smaller amounts and eat the other portion at noon. However, if you eat a large portion in the morning and still want something at noon, eat a salad, a hard-boiled egg or two or even some tuna, or salmon, or sardines.

Don't forget the Supplement at noontime. It is to be taken whether or not you eat lunch. It keeps the apparatus functioning as long as enough protein is still available. By five or six o'clock, you will be ready to supply more protein again. Be sure you take the last Supplement dose for that day, even if you forget and have to take it late. It won't keep you awake. It isn't a stimulant like so many of the appetite suppressors. They really can keep you awake . . . or jittery.

One day, when you have burned up your excess body fat, you no longer will need as much protein, so then you will learn to add some carbohydrates such as bread, milk, even some dessert, but *never as much nor as often as before.* Your intake of carbohydrate while you were gaining weight was too much . . . too often.

If for any reason you decide to discontinue the Supplement at a later date, always remember, you are back to your former igniting level. You must adjust your total intake accordingly.

You won't have to weigh yourself every day, just watch your clothes size. If the clothes that fit you comfortably after you had lost the excess fat begin to feel tight, you don't need the scale to tell you what's happening. Readjust your carbohydrate intake . . . and watch the tightness disappear.

Epilogue

IF the material in this book seems to be repetitious, I intended for it to be so. This is not a novel or mystery story keeping you in suspense until the very last chapter is read. I am trying to deliver a very important message to you and have repeated the key parts in order to make certain that enough of it soaked in. When you read or hear about certain overweights losing a respectable number of pounds . . . how many times have you seen a follow-up on these cases? This brings up the question, what good is losing it if you can't keep it off? I would be little short of unscrupulous if I made claims that all of my patients who have lost weight kept it off. Some persons never change certain habits, and I cannot follow each one personally to forcibly prevent sliding back to deeply-ingrained old patterns. The important fact is that most of the patients that I have guided did . . . and do . . . keep off what they lost. In the final telling it's how you lost that is going to determine the reasonable likelihood of your keeping it off. The Supplement can be continued even after the weight has been lost. Your potential for gaining again is still there. All that is required is an unreasonable increase in carbohydrate intake.

This is my message to you. And now I wish all of you . . . GOOD LOSING.